Surgical Simulation

Surgical Simulation

Edited by Prokar Dasgupta, Kamran Ahmed,
Peter Jaye and Mohammed Shamim Khan

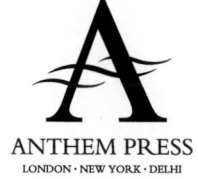

ANTHEM PRESS
LONDON · NEW YORK · DELHI

Anthem Press
An imprint of Wimbledon Publishing Company
www.anthempress.com

This edition first published in UK and USA 2014
by ANTHEM PRESS
75–76 Blackfriars Road, London SE1 8HA, UK
or PO Box 9779, London SW19 7ZG, UK
and
244 Madison Ave #116, New York, NY 10016, USA

© 2014 Prokar Dasgupta, Kamran Ahmed, Peter Jaye
and Mohammed Shamim Khan editorial matter and selection;
individual chapters © individual contributors

The moral right of the authors has been asserted.

All rights reserved. Without limiting the rights under copyright reserved above,
no part of this publication may be reproduced, stored or introduced into
a retrieval system, or transmitted, in any form or by any means
(electronic, mechanical, photocopying, recording or otherwise),
without the prior written permission of both the copyright
owner and the above publisher of this book.

British Library Cataloguing-in-Publication Data
A catalogue record for this book is available from the British Library.

Library of Congress Cataloging-in-Publication Data
Surgical simulation / edited by Prokar Dasgupta, Kamran Ahmed,
Peter Jaye and Mohammed Shamim Khan.
   p. ; cm.
Includes bibliographical references.
ISBN 978-1-78308-156-1 (hbk. ; alk. paper) – ISBN 1-78308-156-2 (hbk. : alk. paper)
I. Dasgupta, Prokar, editor of compilation. II. Ahmed, Kamran, 1977– editor of compilation.
III. Jaye, Peter, 1967– editor of compilation. IV. Khan, Mohammed Shamim, editor of compilation.
   [DNLM: 1. Computer Simulation. 2. General Surgery–education.
      3. Surgical Procedures, Operative–education. WO 18]
            RD29.7
         617.001'13–dc23
            2013047976

ISBN-13: 978 1 78308 156 1 (Hbk)
ISBN-10: 1 78308 156 2 (Hbk)

This title is also available as an ebook.

CONTENTS

1. Surgical Simulation: An Overview — 1
2. Simulation in Historical Perspective: The History of Medical and Surgical Simulation — 15
3. The Role of Animal Models in Surgical Training and Assessment — 23
4. Full Procedural Surgical Simulation — 41
5. Developing Non-technical Skills — 51
6. Learning Curves for Simulators — 63
7. Developing a Simulation Programme — 73
8. Patient Safety and Simulation — 85
9. Psychometrics — 95
10. Future of Surgical Simulation — 111

Author Details — 123

Chapter 1

SURGICAL SIMULATION: AN OVERVIEW

Jason Y. Lee and Elspeth M. McDougall

Simulation-Based Surgical Training

Definitions

Assessment — a process of documenting an individual's knowledge, skills and attitudes or beliefs on a given topic or content

Certification — confirming a specific or pre-determined level of knowledge, skills or attitudes through a formal assessment process

Credentialing — an objective process of establishing the qualifications of individuals or organisations through a formal assessment or evaluative process

Curriculum — any planned educational experience that involves goals, objectives, teaching methods and assessment or evaluation of individuals

Simulation — a person, device, or set of conditions that attempts to imitate a real environment

Virtual reality — a computer-based simulation of a real environment that allows for immersive interaction

As a result of advancements in science and technology, the field of surgery has witnessed significant changes and growth over the past few decades. The introduction of new surgical technologies has also been accompanied by more challenging surgical procedures for a more complex patient population. In addition, factors such as legislated limitations on resident work hours, an increased emphasis on safety and patient-centred care and increasing pressures to utilise costly operating room (OR) resources more efficiently have mandated significant changes to surgical training curricula.

The traditional residency training paradigm established by Dr William Halsted placed a strong emphasis on structured apprenticeships, with trainees developing surgical expertise in a supervised clinical setting over a prolonged training period consisting of increasing levels of responsibility (1). However, the current surgical landscape has required significant modifications to this model, including the development of specific learning objectives outside of the clinical setting and an increased utilisation of simulation-based educational strategies. This repetitive practice of difficult surgical skills in a risk-free environment away from the patient provides the trainee with immediate feedback and the opportunity to train to a predetermined expert proficiency, and seems intuitively, therefore, more efficacious and efficient for both the patient and the healthcare system. This type of surgical education both allows trainees to meet the learning objectives necessary to achieve surgical competency and ensures that they and their surgical educators are able to focus on the development of surgical judgement during the OR experience.

The training of a competent surgeon is, without a doubt, a complex, multi-dimensional process. It is key to any learning activity, however, that the process address three main learning domains relevant to each individual trainee: cognitive, psychomotor and affective objectives (2). In order to meet these learning objectives, it is important to select educational strategies or tools that are congruent with the curricular goals, referred to by educators as a 'goals–tools match'. Simulation-based training is but one such strategy and should be integrated into an overall, well-developed surgical training curriculum. Proponents of simulation must be careful not to anoint it as the panacea for all surgical training issues or deficiencies. For some surgical training objectives, simulation may not provide the requisite experience needed by trainees to achieve competency, no matter how high its fidelity. For other objectives, there may be much simpler and more cost-effective instructional methods that can be utilised to achieve the same educational outcome. It is critical that educators understand the benefits and advantages of simulation-based training over other teaching strategies and implement such methods accordingly, thereby ensuring the 'goals–tools match' so strongly emphasised by contemporary educators (3).

Simulation-based training has been defined as:

> A person, device, or set of conditions which attempts to present evaluation problems authentically. The student or trainee is required to respond to the problems as he or she would under natural circumstances. (4)

While simulation can imitate reality, it does not duplicate real-life clinical situations. Rather than considering this a limitation, it should be viewed as the very reason that simulation-based education can be an effective teaching tool on today's surgical training programmes. One of the key conceptual frameworks relevant to the development of expertise, the theory of deliberate practice (5), espouses the need for multiple repetitions of a skill and the provision of constructive feedback to ensure the skill is being learned correctly. Surgical simulation provides the trainee with an opportunity to repeatedly perform a specific skill, or set of skills, in a low-risk environment away from actual patients, thus allowing for a safe environment where things can 'go wrong' many times over. When properly designed and implemented, simulation-based training methods can also allow for individualised learning that takes into consideration differences in baseline skill levels of the students. There is also the possibility of building different clinical variations into the simulated training sessions, allowing trainees to practise with cases of increasing difficulty and complexity as well as experiencing rare clinical scenarios (6–7). Surgical simulation-based training not only permits structured, comprehensive and immersive learning opportunities, but also allows the educator to provide timely and constructive formative or summative feedback based on trainee performance, ensuring acquisition of correct proficiency-based competency.

Assessment of Trainees Using Surgical Simulation

The ability to provide accurate assessments of students is an essential component of any educational curriculum and is critical to successful surgical residency training (3). Regardless of whether it is the assessment of acquired knowledge and skills, changes in trainee behaviour, modifications to trainee attitudes or the ideal outcome of improved patient care, the ability to provide reliable and valid assessments is of paramount importance, particularly in the case of summative assessments (8–9). Whether it be simulation 'devices' such as pelvic box trainers and virtual reality (VR) laparoscopic simulators, or simulated 'clinical scenarios' such as mock OR team training sessions, surgical simulation-based training methods must be objectively validated and rigorously evaluated if they are to be used for the assessment of trainee competence.

Reliability speaks to the reproducibility of an assessment and is strongly linked to the assessment's validity. It can be estimated by using correlation coefficients, such as Cronbach's alpha, and allows educators to quantify the amount of random error in the measured data, facilitating valid interpretations and the usage of trainee assessment scores. Repeated assessments of a trainee using validated surgical simulators should demonstrate internal consistency with reliability scores of 0.70–0.79 for lower-stake assessments and 0.80–0.89

for moderate-stake assessments, while high-stake assessments, such as certification exams, should demonstrate a reliability of at least 0.90 (10).

Validity evidence for surgical simulation is critical to support any interpretation of assessment data resulting from simulation-based training. Subjective validity evidence includes both face and content validity. While face validity speaks to the 'realism' of the simulator or simulated scenario as judged by non-experts, content validity evidence is provided by content experts who judge the appropriateness of the simulator as a teaching tool. Objective validity evidence is more difficult to obtain but also more robust. Construct validity speaks to the ability of the simulator or simulated scenario to discern the experienced from the novice surgeon. For instance, a robotic surgical simulator with construct validity would reliably discern expert robotic surgeons from novice robotic surgeons by comparing the performance scores of both groups. Concurrent validity is demonstrated if the simulation-based training assessment correlates strongly with assessment data obtained from the accepted 'gold standard' method of determining trainee competence on a particular learning objective. Predictive validity evidence refers to the ability of assessment data obtained during simulation-based training to predict future trainee performance during hands-on clinical surgery (9).

The use of various surgical simulation tools to assess competency, whether for the certification of trainees or the recertification of postgraduate surgeons, requires more than just robust reliability and validity evidence. One of the difficulties in the application of simulation-based tools for assessment purposes is the issue of standard setting: 'establishing credible, defensible, and acceptable passing or cut-off scores […] in health professions education can be challenging' (11). What is the ideal performance score to discern the competent surgical trainee from the incompetent one? What level of performance should be required for certification? Or recertification? These questions must be asked whenever a simulation tool is to be used for assessment purposes.

Standards are usually categorised as either norm-based (relative) or criterion-based (absolute). Norm-based standards determine competency relative to the performance of a well-defined group (e.g., laparoscopic expert surgeons, the top quartile of the class, etc.) and are not ideally suited to high-stakes competency assessments. Criterion-based standards determine trainee competency based on some predetermined absolute level or performance score. As it implies a certain level of mastery of content or skill, criterion-based standards are preferred to assess competency (11). The passing scores for most national specialty certification examinations, for example the American Board of Urology Examinations, are criterion-based.

From De-contextualised to Contextualised Simulation

Along with significant advancements in surgical technology, surgeons have also witnessed considerable advancements in surgical simulation. Technological improvements in simulation fidelity, the increasing integration of valid assessment tools into VR simulators and the improved accessibility of simulation-based training resources have given surgical educators more opportunities to implement a variety of effective surgical simulation tools into contemporary urology training programmes.

Inanimate surgical simulation models range from part-task trainers (e.g., laparoscopic box trainers) to procedure-specific trainers (e.g., ureteroscopy trainers) (Figures 1.1 and 1.2). These synthetic models give trainees the opportunity to deliberately practise a specific surgical skill, or set of skills, in a low-risk environment. Such simulation tools are often ideal for the novice or intermediate trainee, however, due to the lack of clinical variability and the inability to provide individualised, proficiency-based variations in complexity, inanimate surgical simulation models often decrease in utility for advanced-level trainees. In addition, trainee assessments using such synthetic models require significant time and personnel resources from content and/ or education experts. Chapter 3 provides a more comprehensive discussion of the role of synthetic surgical simulation tools in urologic training, both for instructional and assessment purposes.

Animal and cadaveric surgical training models provide improved fidelity and allow the trainee to practise a complete set of technical skills or whole procedures in a context-rich environment. Improved contextual fidelity and the ability to provide procedure-specific training and assessment is offset by the incremental costs associated with these high-fidelity, non-reusable resources. For this reason, it is critical to ensure that the utilisation of animal and cadaveric training models appropriately matches learning objectives and is part of a well-designed, comprehensive curriculum. For example, using animal model training sessions to instruct or assess residents on the basic principles of laparoscopic camera navigation would be a gross misappropriation of resources. An in-depth review of the role of animal and cadaveric models in simulation-based training and assessment in urology is provided in Chapters 4 and 5.

VR flight simulators have been a mainstay of training in the aviation industry for decades, being utilised for instruction, assessment, certification and re-certification purposes. While VR surgical simulators are still relatively rudimentary in comparison to their aviation counterparts, improvements in graphics software, hardware sophistication and built-in performance metrics analytics have significantly improved the fidelity, reliability and validity of modern surgical simulators (Figures 1.3–1.5). Like other simulation-based training tools, VR surgical simulators have the benefit of providing trainees with an opportunity for deliberate practise in a low-risk environment. In addition, clinical variations can be built into the simulator, improving the training content delivered and allowing for individualised, proficiency-based training. The majority of VR surgical simulators currently available also have the advantage of providing instant feedback through analysis of various performance metrics (e.g., time to complete a task, errors committed during a task, instrument motion smoothness and path length or economy of motion). This built-in assessment functionality permits self-directed learning and proficiency-based training, and also removes the necessity of expert faculty presence during the entirety of the training. Despite the improved realism and fidelity of today's VR simulators, rigorous validity evidence is still required for each individual surgical simulator, particularly if it is to be used for competency assessments. The significant cost associated with most endourologic, laparoscopic and robotic surgical simulators also remains a significant obstacle for many training programmes, even further demonstrating the importance of rigorous validation. A detailed review of various VR surgical simulators is provided in Chapter 6.

Attention has increasingly been directed towards the improvement of the non-technical skills of surgical trainees in recent years, as they pertain to the management of crisis OR situations and the overall improvement of patient care. To this end, the development and utilisation of mock OR environments (Figure 1.6) to create high-fidelity simulated clinical scenarios for the purposes of high-reliability team training, crisis OR management training and non-technical skills training and assessment are becoming more commonplace (12, 13). A complete discussion of the use of surgical simulation for the instruction and assessment of interpersonal and communication skills is developed in Chapter 8.

Conclusions

Today's surgical training landscape would likely seem foreign to traditional surgical educators such as Dr William Halsted. Gone are the days of the 'see one, do one, teach one' training paradigm. In an effort to improve patient care outcomes and reduce the impact of surgical training on patient safety, a significant portion of surgical training today is best conducted outside of the clinical OR setting. The growing role of surgical simulation in urological training is supported by the emergence of increasingly robust validity evidence, but educators must be cognisant of the importance of the proper utilisation of surgical simulation as both an instructional and assessment tool. Even the most advanced, high-fidelity simulation tool cannot replace a well-designed, comprehensive training curriculum, nor can it take the place of a well-trained, dedicated surgical educator.

Take-Home Messages

1. Surgical simulation must be integrated into a comprehensive surgical training curriculum and is not a stand-alone training method.
2. Robust reliability and validity evidence is critical to surgical simulation, particularly for the purposes of summative assessment or determination of competency.
3. Surgical simulation provides an opportunity for deliberate practice in a low-risk environment, reducing the footprint of surgical training on patient care outcomes.
4. The ability to incorporate clinical variation and variable levels of difficulty into surgical simulation tools allows for proficiency-based training tailored to the individual trainee.

Figures

Figure 1.1	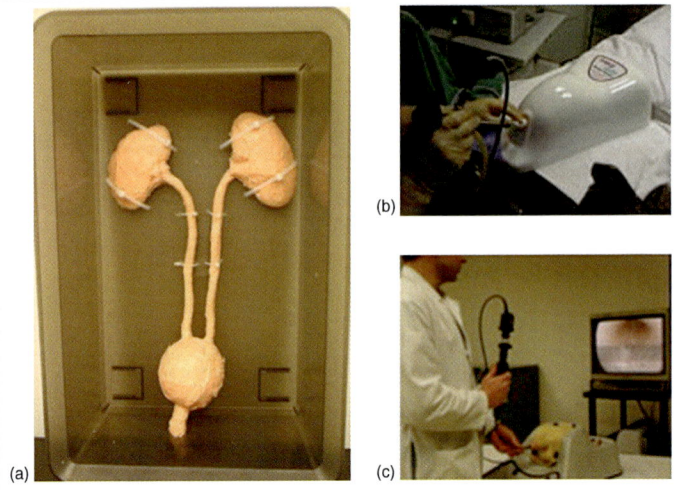
	The silicone KUB model (a) developed at the University of California, Irvine, is a low-cost materials model that allows teaching of the technical skills for cystoscopy, rigid and flexible ureteroscopy and intrarenal surgery. Other commercially available materials models for this same teaching purpose include the Scope Trainer (b) (Mediskills Ltd, Northampton, UK) and Uro-scopic trainer (c) (Limbs & Things Ltd, Bristol, UK).

Figure 1.2	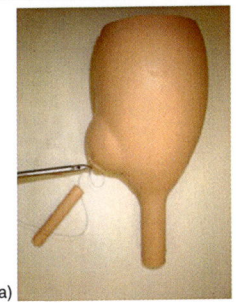 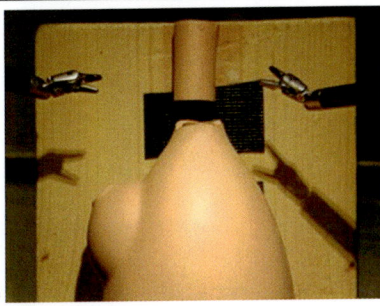 (a) (b) The silicone four-in-one model (Dinsmore & Associates Inc., Costa Mesa, CA) was developed at the University of California, Irvine, to facilitate teaching and practice of the technical skills necessary for laparoscopic or robotic pyeloplasty (a), urethrovesical anastomosis (b), partial nephrectomy and cystorrhaphy.
Figure 1.3	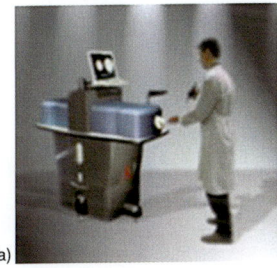 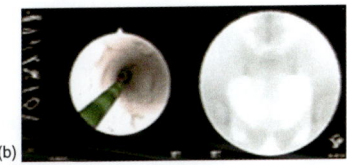 (a) (b) The high-fidelity UroMentor (Simbionix Ltd, Airport City, Israel) is a virtual reality simulator for teaching cystoscopy, ureteroscopy and intrarenal surgery and combines fluoroscopy capability with the endoscopic performance.

Figure 1.4

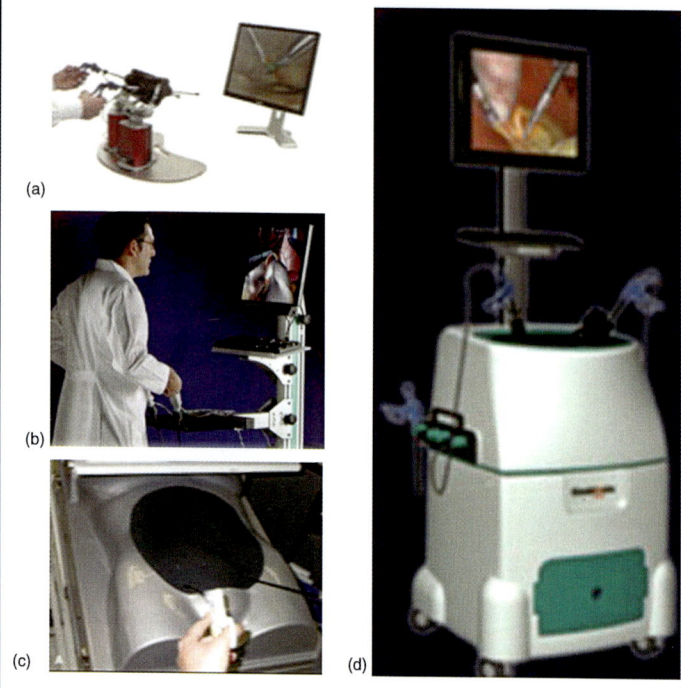

(a)
(b)
(c)
(d)

There are numerous virtual reality laparoscopic surgery simulators available. These can provide basic skills training and procedural skills practice opportunities. Educational learning objectives and cost are the main factors influencing their use in surgical training programmes. None have had rigorous validity testing. Examples here include LapSim (a) (Surgical Science Inc., Goteborg, Sweden), SurgicalSIM (b) (CAE Healthcare, Sarasota, FL), PROMIS simulator (c) (CAE Healthcare, Sarasota, FL), LAP Mentor (d) (Simbionix Ltd, Airport City, Israel).

Figure 1.5

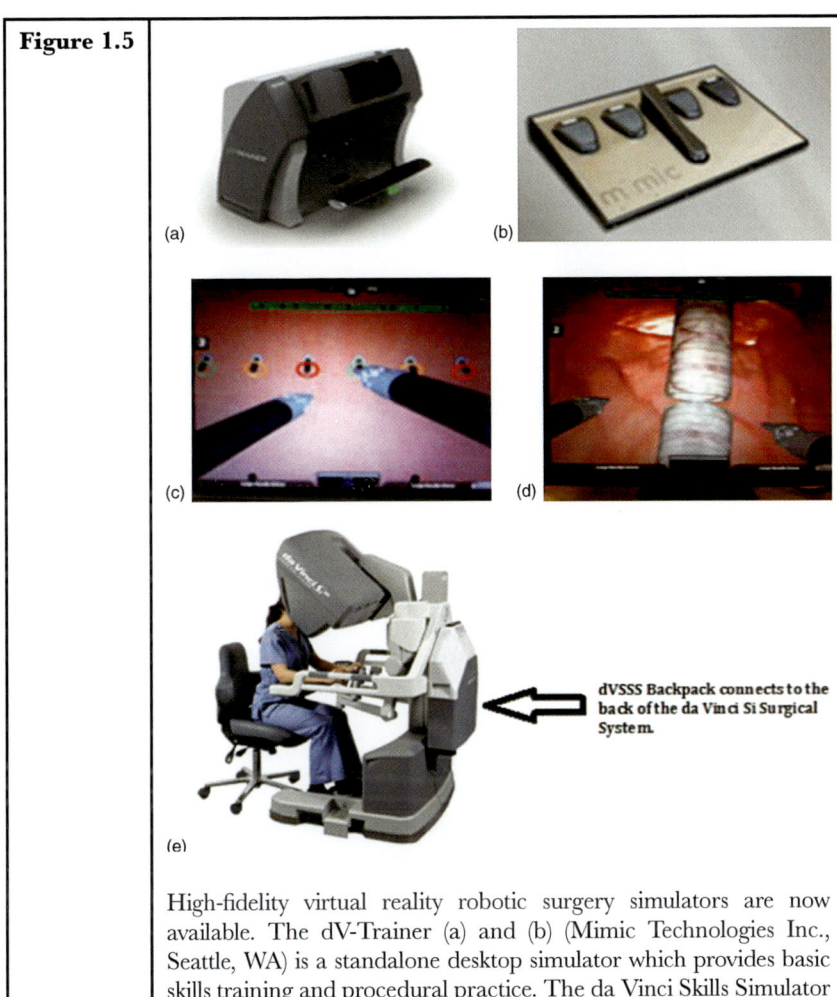

High-fidelity virtual reality robotic surgery simulators are now available. The dV-Trainer (a) and (b) (Mimic Technologies Inc., Seattle, WA) is a standalone desktop simulator which provides basic skills training and procedural practice. The da Vinci Skills Simulator (c) and (d) (Intuitive Surgical Inc., Sunnyvale, CA) consists of the same computer software as the Mimic dV-Trainer but fits as a backpack unit (e) on the clinical Si da Vinci robot (Intuitive Surgical Inc., Sunnyvale, CA).

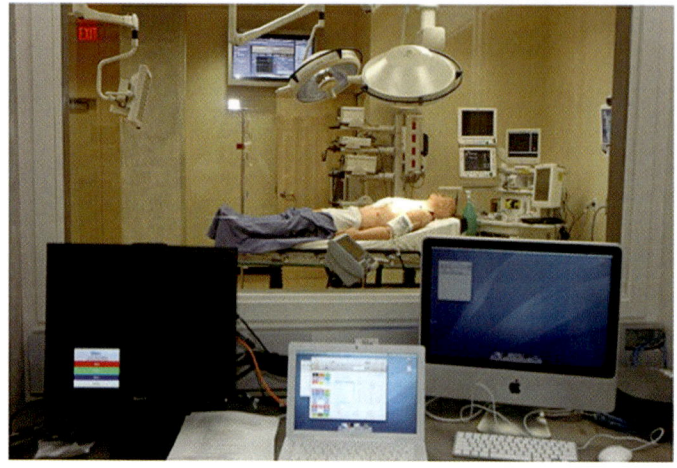

Figure 1.6 University of California, Irvine Medical Education Simulation Center Mock Operating Room with the Human Patient Simulator (CAE Healthcare, Sarasota, FL), OR1 (Karl Storz Endoscopy-America Inc., El Segundo, CA) and one-way glass control desk. A variety of simulation-based team training educational activities are performed in this section of the simulation centre.

References

1. Halsted WS. The training of the surgeon. *Bull Johns Hopkins Hosp.* 1904;15:267–276.
2. Bloom BS. *Taxonomy of Educational Objectives, Handbook 1: The Cognitive Domain.* New York: David McKay; 1956.
3. Kern DE, Thomas PA, Hughes MT. *Curriculum Development for Medical Education: A Six-Step Approach*, second edition. Baltimore: Johns Hopkins University Press; 2009.
4. McGaghie WC. Simulation in professional competence assessment: basic considerations. In: Tekian A, McGuire CH, McGaghie WC, and associates, eds. *Innovative Simulations for Assessing Professional Competence: From Paper-and-Pencil to Virtual Reality.* Chicago: Department of Medical Education, University of Illinois; 1999.
5. Ericsson KA. Deliberate practice and the acquisition and maintenance of expert performance in medicine and related domains. *Acad Med* 2004;79(10):S70–81.
6. Issenberg SB, McGaghie WC, Petrusa ER, Gordon DL, Scalese RJ. Features and uses of high-fidelity medical simulations that lead to effective learning: a BEME systematic review. *Med Teach.* 2005;27(1):10–28.

7. Kneebone R. Evaluating clinical simulations for learning procedural skills: a theory-based approach. *Acad Med.* 2005;80:549–553.
8. Kirkpatrick J, DeWitt-Weaver D, Yeager L. Strategies for evaluating learning outcomes. In: Billings D, Halstead J, eds. *Teaching in Nursing: A Guide to Curriculum, Instruction and Evaluation.* Philadelphia, PA: WB Saunders; 1998.
9. McDougall EM. Validation of Surgical Simulations. *J Endourol.* 2007;21(3):244–247.
10. Downing SM. Reliability: on the reproducibility of assessment data. *Med Educ* 2004;38:1006–1012.
11. Yudkowsky R, Downing SM, Tekian A. Standard setting. In: Downing SM, Yudkowsky R, eds. *Assessment in Health Professions Education.* New York: Routledge; 2009.
12. Lee JY, Mucksavage P, Canales C, McDougall EM, Lin S. High fidelity simulation-based team training in urology: a preliminary interdisciplinary study of technical and nontechnical skills in laparoscopic complications management. *J Urol.* 2012;187(4):1385–1391.
13. Gettman MT, Pereira CW, Lipsky K, Wilson T, Arnold JJ, Leibovich BC, et al. Use of high fidelity operating room simulation to assess and teach communication, teamwork, and laparoscopic skills: initial experience. *J Urol.* 2009;181(3):1289–1296.

Chapter 2

SIMULATION IN HISTORICAL PERSPECTIVE: THE HISTORY OF MEDICAL AND SURGICAL SIMULATION

Ali Nehme Bahsoun, Sarah Wheatstone and Ben Challacombe

Introduction

The word 'simulate' was originally derived from the Latin term *simulare* (to imitate) stemming from *similis* (similar), and therefore to simulate is to create likeness or to model (1). Simulation itself has been defined as 'in industry, science, and education, a research or teaching technique that reproduces actual events and processes under test conditions' (2). Simulation can include many activities such as clay pigeon shooting, practising fire drills or exercising on rowing machines. Surgical simulation itself can be defined as 'an exercise that reproduces or emulates, under artificial conditions, components of surgical procedures that are likely to occur under normal circumstances' (3).

Historical Overview

The aim of simulation is to aid the acquisition of specific skills and improve both competence and confidence. When we hear the term 'simulation' today we are likely to imagine the fully immersive high-fidelity simulators training airline pilots or astronauts, however, simulation has been a part of training for thousands of years, from hunter-gatherers throwing wooden spears while learning to hunt to target archers using the bow and arrow. In surgical training, using an orange to practise suturing skills or practising surgical knots on a table leg are methods of simulation that have been employed for many years.

Perhaps the earliest contribution to the field of surgical simulation was by the ancient Indian surgeon, Sushruta Samhita (4). As well as describing over

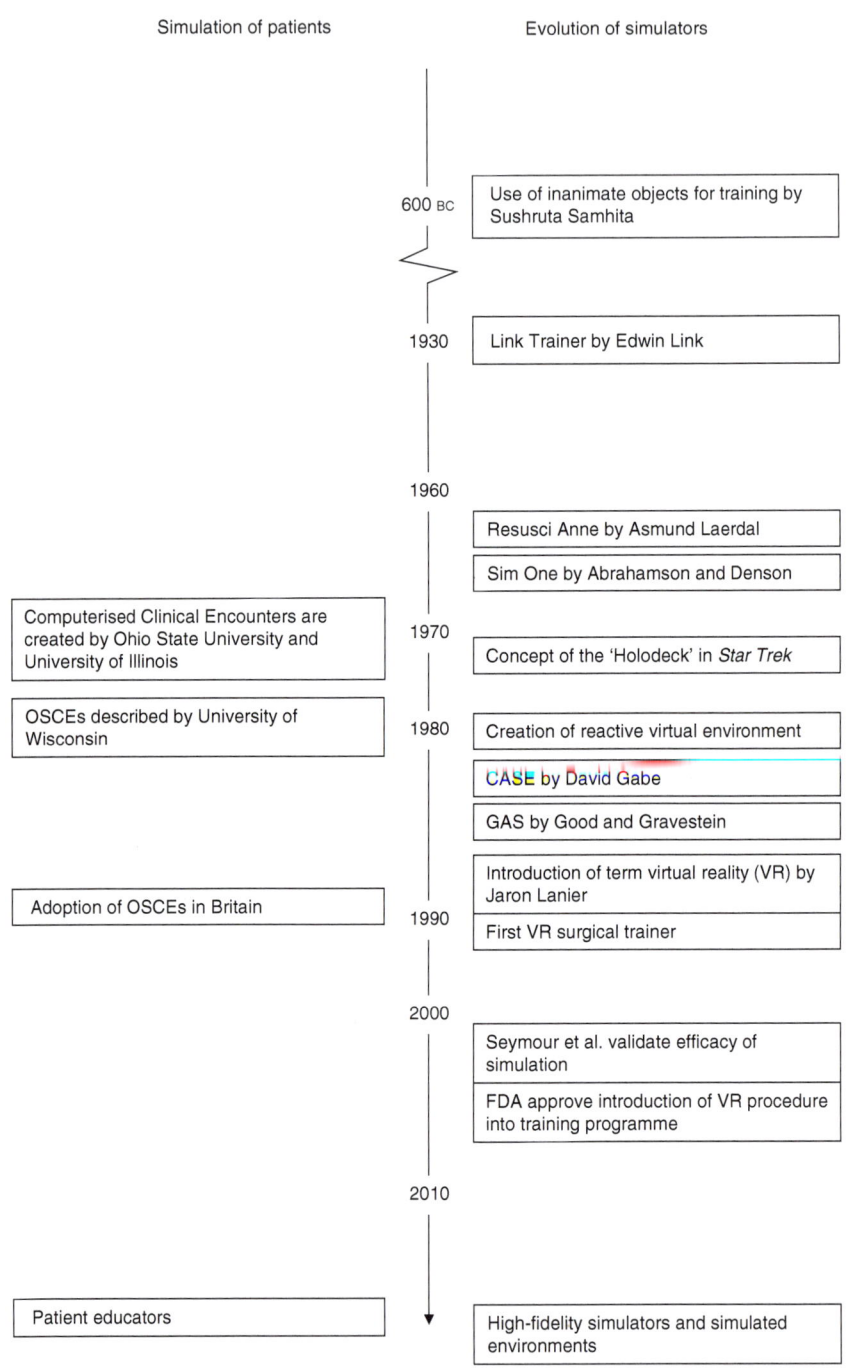

120 surgical instruments and 300 operations in his surgical treatise written around 2,600 years ago, he was arguably the earliest to have advocated operative practice on inanimate objects. Within an apprenticeship model, Sushruta advocated the use of cadavers and synthetic models for practice prior to surgery. He taught technical skills using experimental modules that included probing on worm-eaten wood and incising into vegetables such as watermelons, gourds and cucumbers.

In the fourth century BC Plato believed that medicine should be considered a science and thus should be taught through observation and experience. Hippocrates believed that a good doctor was one who aimed to impress their patients with confidence and would also call upon the sound knowledge of disease pathology and management as a great tool to demonstrate competence (5). In more modern times, William Halsted's concept of training in surgery is summarised by the famous phrase, 'see one and do one and teach one'. Simulation, however, challenges this whole Halstedian ethos of surgical training that has been widely used over the last century.

Until 2003, the UK-based surgical training system, like most others around the world, was founded on a traditional apprenticeship model with a basis that had not changed significantly throughout several millennia. Surgical students learned their trade by observation and assisting in the treatment of their masters' patients. It was taken upon the student to recognise patterns, to devise theories for their patients' ailments and plan treatments with the aid of their experience, texts and teachers, and learn technical skills through observation and mentoring. Apprenticeships demanded that surgeons seek out their career path from an early stage and persevere with it. The Hippocratic texts had claimed that, 'he who aspires to practise surgery must go to war' and that truly if you wished to learn something then you had to immerse yourself in it (5).

Nowadays we work within strict time regulations limiting the amount of training hours and medical education is based on yearly progression through competencies, thus the real clinical environment may not provide the student or trainee with sufficient opportunity to build up their skills or confidence to the required level. It is also impossible to guarantee a uniform clinical experience at various different hospitals, and thus medical students turn to lectures, textbooks, web sources and, increasingly, simulation. This new system has moved away from apprenticeships and called for an integrated system of electronic training aids assisting trainees through a curriculum. This new system has opened the doors for surgical simulation to flourish in the UK and, as we have seen, using simulation to accelerate skill acquisition is not a new concept (6). The current tools available for simulation can be broken down into the following four areas: simulator models, simulated patients, training tissues and virtual reality.

The Evolution of Simulation Models

The first modern skills 'simulator' was produced in 1928 when Edwin Link created a pilot trainer. The trainer consisted of a pilot seat mounted on a pedestal that could pitch, roll, dive and climb. The Link Trainer allowed trainee pilots to learn important aeronautical manoeuvres whilst remaining on the ground, making learning to fly cheaper, safer and more accessible. Three years after the creation of the Link Trainer, the army bought six trainers and this number had grown to 6,271 by the end of WWII (7).

One of the earliest examples of medical simulation was a foetal model and human pelvis bone used by Madame du Coudray to train midwives in eighteenth-century France (8). The first widespread medical simulator was built in 1960 when a girl who drowned in the River Seine in Paris inspired Asmund S. Laerdal, a toy maker, to create a resuscitation training manikin. The mouth to mouth training aid was made to look realistic and life-sized in the hope that it would be more motivating for students to treat the situation as if it were real. Laerdal had even fashioned the face of his training device into the face of the drowned victim. Laerdal's mouth to mouth simulator became the Resusci Anne and is still widely used today by first aid courses and life support training. The Resusci Anne was built to be low-cost, thus making it readily available, and since its creation others have developed a variety of models with an increasing complexity and number of uses (9).

Later in the 1960s, a more sophisticated trainer was developed by Abrahamson and Denson called Sim One. This device could simulate breathing, heart rate, pulses and blood pressure, and had eyes and a mouth that could open and close. Sim One proved to be very good at what it did, however the medical profession was still fixated on learning through apprenticeship on real patients so it was not widely adopted at the time. High-fidelity training would not be revisited until the 1980s, which gave rise to two notable devices. The first of the two was known as the Comprehensive Anaesthetic Simulation Environment (CASE) and was built by a group led by David Gaba at Stanford University. CASE used the concept of a team-based realistic environment adapted from the aviation training model of crew resource management to teach anaesthetic crisis management from the anaesthetics curriculum. The second, the Gainesville Anaesthetic Simulator (GAS), was developed by a team led by Michael Good and J. S. Gravenstein at the University of Florida. CASE would later become Medsim and GAS became Medical Education Technologies. The movement towards high-fidelity training was led primarily by anaesthetists. Since the conception of CASE and GAS, high-fidelity training has seen a steady rise in its adoption in the medical curriculum (10).

Today, high-fidelity training focuses on the technical and non-technical skills required to make a good doctor and also adds an encompassing realistic environment to simulation scenarios. Modern simulation centres include artificial wards, GP surgeries and operating theatres and even the 'igloo', an inflatable surgical environment with posters of typical theatre equipment. The use of these environments in simulation is known as 'immersive training'.

Simulated Patients

Medical education has also adopted the use of people and computers to simulate doctor–patient encounters. The first computerised simulator for clinical encounters was created in 1970 in Massachusetts General Hospital and soon afterwards sponsorships were made for access to medical simulation at Ohio State University and the University of Illinois (10).

By 1973, the University of Wisconsin had developed their own patient encounter simulator, which later became the basis for computerised examinations, and two years later objective structured clinical examinations (OSCEs) were first described.

By using OSCEs the training institutions could simulate a standardised situation or environment that would require the student or trainee to demonstrate their competence and confidence. In the 1990s, OSCEs were adopted by many divisions of healthcare education within British universities and they still play a huge role in examining students and trainees today (11).

Simulated patients have also taken on the role of teaching as well as testing students and trainees. Institutions currently use actors and real patients to work with students as 'student educators' and help them develop their communication and examination skills. The use of patients in the education of future doctors is also helping to develop patient-centred healthcare as the public are gaining the chance to influence how students communicate with future patients (12).

Patient educators also have a great role in helping students through sensitive topics and examinations such as the cervical smear and bimanual vaginal examination. King's College London runs a scheme whereby 'gynaecology training associates' (GTAs) are trained to teach students using their own bodies as an educational tool. When asked about GTAs, students have used comments such as, 'GTAs are very supportive; they help you use the right words, how to behave in a professional yet caring manner. I feel very confident now if I had to do a VE or smear test' (13).

Training Tissue and Models

Today, 2,600 years after Sushruta, medical and surgical training has still maintained the use of basic training materials. Oranges and bananas have become more than just food to medical students, being their suture trainers too. Current synthetic models have greatly improved in look, feel and tactile behaviour and many medical device companies now produce a huge range of general and specialist surgical skills models from high-fidelity materials. The use of animal and cadaveric models to simulate real surgery has also been in practice for many years, but there are considerable costs in setting up and running these modes of training. Despite this, the use of cadavers has been increasingly adopted in medical education and skills courses by the British Royal Colleges. Furthermore, the Cruelty to Animals Act of 1876 makes it illegal to use live animals for surgical training in the UK.

Virtual Reality Training

The perfect training tool would be one that can combine simulation, immersion and interaction. The earliest combination of these three attributes was in Gene Roddenberry's fictional 'Holodecks' in *Star Trek*, which were inspired by the work of the holographer and inventor of the digital projector, Gene Dologoff. Holodecks were rooms created for training, event recreation and scientific experimentation and were first shown in 1973 on *Star Trek: The Animated Series*. They used holographs, force fields and matter to fulfil their functions (14, 15).

In the late 1970s, this concept became a reality when stereoscopic video goggles and fibre-optic data gloves were adopted to create computer-generated environments which responded to the user. The experience of using such a device was later given the term 'virtual reality' (VR) in 1989 by Jaron Lanier, an American computer scientist. Lanier had taken the concept of 'virtual', describing something that appeared to exist without actually existing such as virtual memory, from the 1960s, and combined it with the term 'reality', meaning something that is observable and measurable as opposed to the imaginary or delusional (16).

In 1990 Delp et al. developed the first VR surgical simulator with a view to teaching lower limb reconstruction surgery, and by the late 1990s medical virtual reality models had reached the widespread commercial market (17). Concerns over their efficacy were put to rest after a double-blinded trial was published in 2002 by Seymour et al. showing that trainees could significantly reduce their procedure times to perform a cholecystectomy by 29% and were five times less likely to injure the gallbladder after using a VR trainer (18).

In 2004 the Federal Food and Drug Administration (FDA) in America approved the introduction of the VR carotid stent procedure into their training programme. For the first time trainees had to prove themselves on a competency-based task to be allowed to perform a real procedure (19).

Now virtual reality trains not only surgeons as newer simulations include virtual reality patients, built on the concept of the simulated patient, and even virtual reality therapists for patients. The future of medical and surgical education does not solely lie with one form of simulation but in the combination of different modalities being integrated into the curriculum. With time we can expect more complex and advanced devices, however our main drive should be returning to Asmund Laerdal's concept of cheap and accessible training. In time, we may witness a shift in where trainees conduct their own web-based simulation, as the web has already proven itself to be a great place for cheap and accessible resources. With huge interest surrounding the impact of video games on surgical aptitude, we might also see the uptake of video games as a platform for surgical simulation.

References

1. Dictionary.com. Simulation. http://dictionary.reference.com/browse/simulation. Accessed 12 December 2012.
2. Dictionary.com. Simulate. http://dictionary.reference.com/browse/simulate. Accessed 12 December 2012.
3. Krummel TM. Surgical simulation and virtual reality: the coming revolution. *Ann Surg.* 1998;228:635–637.
4. Das S. Urology in ancient India. *Indian J Urol.* 2007;23:2–5.
5. Pikoulis E, et al. Evolution of medical education in Ancient Greece. *Chin Med J.* 2008;121(21):2202–2206.
6. Medical education in the UK: building a firm foundation. *Lancet.* 2005;366(9486):607.
7. Stark Ravings. The Link Trainer. http://www.starksravings.com/linktrainer/linktrainer.htm. Accessed 12 December 2012.
8. Ker J, Bradley P. *Simulation in Medical Education.* Edinburgh: Association for the Study of Medical Education; 2007.
9. Laerdal. The girl from the River Seine. http://www.laerdal.com/gb/docid/1117082/The-Girl-from-the-River-Seine. Accessed 12 December 2012.
10. Bradley P. The history of simulation in medical education and possible future directions. *Med Educ.* 2006;40(3):254–262.

11. OSCE Home. What is OCSE? http://www.oscehome.com/What_is_Objective-Structured-Clinical-Examination_OSCE.html. Accessed 12 December 2012.
12. King's College London. Patient educators. http://www.kcl.ac.uk/medicine/research/divisions/meded/innovation/educators.aspx. Accessed 12 December 2012.
13. King's College London. Gynaecology and breast teaching associates. http://www.kcl.ac.uk/medicine/research/divisions/meded/innovation/associate.aspx. Accessed 14 December 2012.
14. Wikipedia. Holodeck. http://en.wikipedia.org/wiki/Holodeck. Accessed 15 December 2012.
15. Wikipedia. Star Trek: The Animated Series. http://en.wikipedia.org/wiki/Star_Trek:_The_Animated_Series. Accessed 15 December 2012.
16. Ebersole S. A brief history of virtual reality and its social applications. http://faculty.colostate-pueblo.edu/samuel.ebersole/336/eim/papers/vrhist.html. Published 1997. Accessed 16 December 2012.
17. Delp SL, Loan JP, Hoy MG, Zajac FE, Topp EL, Rosen JM. An interactive graphics-based model of the lower extremity to study orthopaedic surgical procedures. *IEEE Trans Biomed Eng.* 1990;37:757-767.
18. Seymour NE, Gallagher AG, Roman SA, et al. Virtual reality training improves operating room performance: results of a randomized, double-blinded study. *Ann Surg.* 2002;236:458-463.
19. Scerbo, BMW. Medical virtual reality simulators: have we missed an opportunity? *Bulletin by Human Factors and Ergonomics Society.* 2005; 48(5):1–7.

Chapter 3

THE ROLE OF ANIMAL MODELS IN SURGICAL TRAINING AND ASSESSMENT

Lars Lund and Johan Poulsen

Abstract

Simulation is of paramount importance to practising skills, problem solving and judgement, and animal models provide the cornerstone of this method. Research advocates a combination of training with bench and animal models and simulation. The animal model used most often is the pig because its anatomy is very similar to humans'. In research, mice, rats and rabbits are largely used because they are easier to handle and less costly.

The training and implementation of minimally invasive surgery demands extensive resources. The most realistic way to train and observe trainees in specific procedures is by using animal-based models due to the realistic nature of their tissue and blood flow. It is important that the trainee masters basic procedures, some of which include positioning the patient, becoming familiar with instrumentation and understanding the potential complications of the operation peri-operatively. All this can be learned in a wet lab in a quiet atmosphere. Wet lab training may also be utilised for the selection of potential trainees and when offering careers to junior doctors.

During the last decade many wet laboratories have opened and many commercial companies have started to run courses in well-equipped, high-tech laboratories with state-of-the-art instrumentation available. In addition, it is important that hospitals are well equipped and involved in simulation in order to offer local training.

It is essential that future studies focus on the design and validation of training models and a comprehensive curriculum for the training and assessment of cognitive, technical and non-technical components. This will provide tools to define the learning curve for easy and difficult procedures.

Background on Animal Models

Medical simulation is 'an imitation of some real thing or process', and the historical roots of simulation for practising skills, problem solving and judgement are well known (1). Practice is important to learn and maintain skills. Innovations in flight simulation, resuscitation, technology and plastics were essential antecedents to medical simulation, which began at the end of the twentieth century and is recognised as a major step in the evolution of health science education (2).

David Gaba describes the five categories of simulation as verbal, standardised patients (SP), part-task trainers, computer patients and electronic patients (1). Verbal simulation is simply role-playing. SP are actors used to educate and evaluate history taking and physical examination skills, communication and professionalism. Part-task trainers may be simple anatomical models of body parts in their normal state or representing a disease. The more complex modern surgical task trainers are also included in this category. Computer patients are interactive and may be software-based or part of an internet-based virtual world. These patients serve the same functions as SP in many areas at a reduced cost. The most comprehensive form of simulation is the electronic patient. Electronic patients can be either manikin or VR-based, and replication of the clinical environment is integral (3). Simulations also use other materials, such as animals and cadavers. In 1959, a cardiovascular simulator for the evaluation of prosthetic aortic valves was described, however the first manikin-based systems appeared in the 1960s and an anaesthesia simulation to recreate the operating room environment appeared in 1988 (4, 5).

It is important to state that animal models have a higher degree of face validity but their use is limited by several factors including cost, ethical considerations, logistics, animal licenses and lack of pathological conditions. Increasingly, more complex simulation systems are being developed for surgical training, whilst isolating and measuring skills in the simulator that translate to the operating room has become more difficult. We advocate that there should be a combination of training with bench and animal models and simulation. However, the most realistic way to train and examine trainees in specific procedures is to utilise animal models, e.g., pigs, due to their realistic tissue and vascular properties. It is important that the trainee masters the basic procedures, some of which may include positioning the patient, becoming familiar with instrumentation and understanding the potential complications of the operation peri-operatively. All this can be learned in a wet lab with a quiet atmosphere. Wet lab training may also be utilised for the selection of potential trainees and when offering careers to junior doctors.

Types of Animal Models

There are many different training methods such as didactic training, skills training (dry lab, virtual reality, animal or cadaveric models), case observation, bedside assisting, proctoring in laparoscopy and the mentoring console for training in robotics-assisted laparoscopic surgery. Several general and specific training programmes described in surgical literature are designed for residents, fellows and surgeons.

The animal model used most often is the pig in urological training. The anatomy of the pig is very similar to that of the human. In research, mice, rats, and rabbits are used most often because they are easier to handle and less costly. There are several wet lab programmes training in different scenarios, with models made from animal tissue for open surgery and live anaesthetised animals for laparoscopy (see Tables 3.1 and 3.2).

Evidence for the Effectiveness of Animal Model Training

The scientific evidence monitoring the effectiveness of animal training is growing. A new programme has just been described and validated which combines simulator and wet lab training (6). The study concluded that a centralised simulation programme would be expected to improve the performance of future surgeons and thus improve patient safety. Whether it would affect learning curves and operating times compared to conventional procedures is still a matter of debate. Nowadays there are numerous possibilities for learning laparoscopic techniques including pelvitrainers and virtual reality computer programs. One useful and realistic way involves wet lab training programmes for ablative and reconstructive procedures using the pig model. In addition, laparoscopy in urological surgery includes procedures with low- (e.g., laparoscopy for undescended testicles), intermediate- (laparoscopic pyeloplasty) and high- (laparoscopic/endoscopic prostatectomy) level complexity. Laparoscopy should be an integral part of training in urology. There are a number of national and international training centres with structured educational programmes, and it is mandatory to have standardised surgical procedures as well as educational training programmes in order to shorten individual learning curves and generate common quality standards to minimise patient risk. An example of this is the 'Hospital das Clinicas' of the Sao Paulo Medical School which offers a laparoscopic training programme for urological residents in both dry and wet lab environments. It performed a critical analysis of the cost–benefit ratio of an advanced laparoscopic skills laboratory involving two virtual simulators, three manual simulators and four laparoscopic sets for study with a porcine model. During their first year, urology residents attend classes in the virtual and manual simulators and help the senior urological resident in activities carried out with the laparoscopic sets. During the second year, urological residents have six periods per week, each lasting four hours, to perform laparoscopic procedures with a porcine model. In a training programme of ten weeks, each urological resident performs an average of 120 urological procedures. The most common procedures are total nephrectomy (30%), bladder suture (30%), partial nephrectomy (10%), pyeloplasty (10%), ureteral replacement or transuretero anastomosis (10%) and others like adrenalectomy, prostatectomy, and retroperitoneoscopy (7). Better quality studies are needed to define the learning curve for easy and difficult procedures. It is essential that future studies should focus on the design and validation of training models, and on a comprehensive curriculum for the training and assessment of cognitive, technical and non-technical components of competency for laparoscopic surgery. A new study reviewed the training for laparoscopic Roux-en-Y gastric bypass (LRYGBP) (8). The aim was to see whether ex vivo simulation-based technical skills training improved operating room performance and shortened the learning curves for basic laparoscopic procedures. They found 12 studies involving bench-top laparoscopic jejunojejunostomy, anaesthetised animals and Thiel human cadavers made up the bulk of the reported models for ex vivo training. Most studies were of relatively poor quality. They concluded that an evidence-based ex vivo training curriculum for LRYGBP is currently lacking feasibility, validity and educational impact.

Courses Available

During the last decade many wet labs have opened and many commercial companies have arranged courses in well-equipped, high-tech laboratories with new instruments available. However, it is also important that hospitals at different levels are involved in this in order to offer local training (see Table 3.3 for available courses).

Cost Implications

It is very expensive to run a wet lab. One has to invest in and build an operating room with all relevant instruments available, e.g., laparoscopic stack, theatre table and equipment for anaesthesia, etc. Besides this, a secretary must be in place to take care of the logistics and keep in contact with trainees, trainers and different departments. Also, education materials including PowerPoint presentations, leaflets, etc. have to be formed. The lab has to have a well-educated staff, e.g. technicians and veterinarians, in order to take care of the animals during an operation. The annual cost of running the Danish MIDC, not including investments in equipment or buildings, is approximately 500,000 euros.

How to Set Up Training Centres for Animal Model Training

Today, laparoscopic urological surgery includes procedures with low- (e.g., laparoscopy for undescended testicles), intermediate- (laparoscopic pyeloplasty) and high-level (laparoscopic/endoscopic prostatectomy) complexity. Laparoscopy should be an integral part of training in urology. There are a number of national and international training centres with well structured educational programmes. It is mandatory to have standardisation of surgical procedures as well as educational training programmes in order to shorten individual learning curves and generate common quality standards minimising patient risks. The Danish MIDC model is another example of how to set up a wet lab.

The MIDC Model (Minimally Invasive Development Centre)

In 2005 a 'brick-less' (virtual) minimally invasive development centre (MIDC) was created among the regional hospitals of western Denmark to secure a standardised level of training for the next generation of laparoscopic surgeons (10). The success of this new programme is ensured by three guiding principles: (i) surgery, gynaecology and urology have common basic theoretical concepts; (ii) collaboration between the specialties to ensure innovation in education; and (iii) continuous research to evaluate the programme and the quality of training. Specifically, a structured modular laparoscopic skills course that encompasses the principles of self-directed as well as guided learning has been developed (11). This course is intended to facilitate the development of laparoscopic dexterity in the junior trainee, and with additional training it is possible to improve laparoscopic operative performance significantly. To the best of our knowledge this approach has not been used elsewhere in Denmark or abroad. Following this programme, the trainee can gain high-level skills before operating on real patients in the operating theatre. These improvements can be accomplished in a cost-effective curriculum that is intended to enhance the surgical education of residents.

In an initial assessment of regional programmes, the variation in the quality of education directed at teaching laparoscopy was large. Although there were several bench-top simulators at all the regional hospitals as well as three experimental virtual reality laparoscopic simulators and three surgical animal laboratories, the format of education, including the curriculum, had not been standardised throughout the network. In response to this variation, a steering committee with members of the different surgical specialties was called to ensure the strategic development and implementation of a standardised, simulation-based training programme.

In response to a clearly articulated need, the MIDC purchased portable laparoscopic trainers (transportable 'black boxes', LiNA Medical ApS, Denmark) to facilitate the independent practice of technical skills in the early stages of learning. Trainees were encouraged to borrow and take home the portable trainers to practise independently before the part of the course guided by experts. In addition, the trainees received a package with reading material, access to relevant websites and a CD-ROM with expert instruction on various laparoscopic exercises. This concept is novel to the programme and its efficacy is currently being experimentally evaluated. The expert-guided learning format consists of four modules. Module 1 (Figure 3.1) is a two-day course in which all the trainees receive expert guidance on their performance of a skill set previously practised independently. Their technical performance before and after the module is objectively assessed to provide the trainee with feedback. Module 2 (Figures 3.2–3.4) is a three-day animal course, teaching advanced procedures and including a CD-ROM with expert demonstrations of the operations the trainees will be performing. This module also covers the evaluation and certification of technical skills before and after training. The next step in this programme, in cooperation with the society of each specialty, is the development of Modules 3 and 4, which involves the implementation of a logbook system that records details of actual procedures assisted, supervised and performed. It should be mentioned that there are many other national and international wet labs, e.g., at Newcastle, Dundee and the Royal Colleges in the UK, as well as Strasbourg, Hamburg, Amsterdam, Paris and Toronto (see Table 3.3).

Evolution

Currently, the field of laparoscopic surgery is facing a problem shared by several other surgical subspecialties: how to deliver the initial phases of training in laparoscopic procedures safely and adequately to the next generation of surgeons. As surgical education becomes more evidence based by addressing learning theory in the development of training regimens, there is a growing need for mentors with a background in educational science, skilled in the effective delivery of knowledge, and who recognise the needs of individual trainees in order to ensure a supportive environment for acquiring skills (12). Because of the improved clinical outcomes, increasingly, many patients are choosing to be treated laparoscopically. However, urological societies (e.g., in Denmark and the UK) have faced difficulties in training the new generation of urologists in laparoscopic surgical approaches because there are so few surgeons available to mentor laparoscopic training. The British Association of Urological Surgeons (BAUS) has presented guidelines for urological laparoscopic training in the UK (13). According to these guidelines, the training of laparoscopic urologists should be rooted in simulation and augmented by intraoperative experience. Specifically, these guidelines suggest that training should combine the 'hands-on' practice of basic laparoscopic skills (practice on low- and high-fidelity bench models, assisting in and observing various laparoscopic urological procedures) with an advanced skills course (operative experience on cadaver or animal models) rather than relying solely on a logbook system that records the numbers of procedures performed or assisted (14).

Effective simulation-based training must consist of three elements: the simulator(s), the curriculum (with validated assessment methods) and the educator. Accordingly, BAUS provides adequate guidelines for two of these three components and states that centres with bigger numbers report better outcomes (15).

Effectiveness of Courses

In the MIDC model more than 200 young doctors have now passed Modules 1 and 2. We have made a report on this concept focusing on 106 trainees who were non-specialised doctors from a specific region in Denmark (10). They underwent theoretical and practical specialised training in laparoscopy in the period 2006–2008. The training had several modules of which the first two are described. The training and evaluation methods used were objective and structured tests (OSCE test) and objective skill assessments tests (OSATS test). Of the 106 trainees, a total of 80 passed. In Module 1, the distribution of participants with regard to speciality was: surgery, 47, urology, 14 and gynaecology, 45. Six trainees were not certified. We have registered OSATS scores for 64 participants with a median score of 3.0 (range 1–4.4). To pass the multiple choice test, participants needed to answer 66% of the questions correctly. Twenty participants out of 57 (35%) were below this level in Module 1 and 32 out of 60 (53%) in Module 2.

In the practical part, a group of 6% could not achieve the sufficient level of certification. It has previously been suggested that there is a group of about 10% who have limited learning abilities for laparoscopy simulation (16). The OSATS test is a recognised validation method. We have chosen certification level 1.7 as it shows that the student has progressed from the 1.0 baseline. Because the minimally invasive approach in future surgery is expected to incorporate all types of operations, it makes little sense to train doctors for surgery without learning endoscopy and laparoscopy. Since the literature has very convincingly documented that there is consistency between simulator performance and real surgery, colleagues who have limited learning ability on simulator training should be encouraged to take up a non-surgical specialty. A proposal for training in the skills lab is presented here together with the first Danish attempt at systematic certification in laparoscopic skills. The majority of students will in the course of five intensive training days gain sufficient skills to move forward to human operations. A small minority will need additional training (20%) and even fewer will not pass the tests (5%). These figures are further investigated in one of the programmes of a PhD student supported by MIUD. The clinical effects of this training now remain to be evaluated in the form of improved outcomes in theatres and on wards. Also, the trainees' attitudes towards surgical training and factors that improve a flat learning curve should be identified. Our study suggests that simulator training probably could be a tool that helps in the selection of possible candidates for surgical training posts (17). In a recent Cochrane review all randomised clinical studies in the field were analysed to discover whether simulation (virtual reality simulation) could replace conventional laparoscopic training (18). The study included 23 individual studies (simulation over other forms of exercise: black box, no training or standard laparoscopic training with a total of 612 participants). The conclusion was that simulation could replace conventional learning and was actually better than black box exercises.

Conclusion

The future of surgery depends on novel training tools which match highly sophisticated operating techniques. The continued partnership of training and clinical practice is necessary to ensure that these innovations are translated to the operating room so benefits to patients can be maximised. Training and implementation in minimally invasive surgery demands resources. However, the most realistic way to train in specific procedures and observe the trainees is in through animal models, e.g., pigs, due to the realistic tissue handling and blood flow. It is important that the trainee learns the procedure from the beginning, with the planning phase, positioning of the patient, which instruments should be used and how, and risk and complications during and after the operation. All this can be learned in a wet lab with a quiet atmosphere. Training in the wet lab may also be used for the selection of trainees when advice regarding future career choices is given.

Figures and Tables

Table 3.1. Laparoscopic training on live animal models – a three-day intermediate level course for general surgery, gynaecology and urology specialist registrars

Day 1	
08:15–08:30	Introduction
08:30–09:30	Therorectical lectures: • Planning and preparation in laparoscopic surgery • Quality assessment • Complications in laparoscopic urology • Golden rules of laparoscopic surgery
09:30–15:30	Live surgery on animal models – learning by doing: • Establishing pneumoperitoneum – different methods • Diagnostic laparoscopy • Laparoscopic cholecystectomy
15:30–16:00	Reznik evaluation of trainees by the trainers (global rating scale)
Day 2	
08:15–09:00	Lecture on pathophysiological issues during laparoscopic surgery
09:00–15:30	Surgery on live animal models: • Appendicectomy • Side-to-side anastomosis using suturing and staplers
15:30–16:00	Reznik evaluation of each trainee by the trainers
Day 3	
08:15–08:45	Multiple choice test
08:45–12:00	Final Reznik evalution of every trainee performing a lap. cholecystectomy, lap. appendicectomy or bowel side-to-side anastomosis (global rating scale)
12:00–15:00	Laparoscopic nephrectomy on live animal model
15:00–16:00	Individual debriefing and evaluation of each trainee (multiple choice test and Reznik scheme)

Table 3.2. Advanced training course in laparoscopic urology – a one-day course, 07:30–16:00

Morning
Handling of laparoscopic instruments
Insertion and removal of laparoscopic ports
Retroperitoneoscopy using a dilating balloon
Left simulated ureterolithotomy
Left retroperitoneoscopic nephrectomy
Afternoon
Laparoscopic cholecystectomy
Laparoscopic bladder repair
Laparoscopic pelvic lymph node dissection
Laparoscopic radical prostatectomy
Laparoscopic lower pole resection of the right kidney using the ultrascision device
Transperitoneal right nephrectomy
Laparoscopic handling of vascular incidents

Table 3.3. European laparoscopic surgery training courses

Course name	Location	Webpage link	Type	Notes
Laparoscopic psychomotor skills	European Academy of Gynaecological Surgery, Leuven, Belgium	http://www.europeanacademy.org	N/A	Offers LASTT training package
A–Z laparoscopic suturing	European Academy of Gynaecological Surgery, Leuven, Belgium	http://www.europeanacademy.org	Dry lab / wet lab	
Transvaginal laparoscopy course	European Academy of Gynaecological Surgery, Leuven, Belgium	http://www.europeanacademy.org	Dry lab	
Minimal access surgery	Minimal Access Therapy Training Unit, University of Surrey, United Kingdom	http://www.mattu.org.uk/	Dry lab / wet lab	Offers 60 courses annually
EITS surgical courses	European Institute of TeleSurgery, Strasbourg, France	http://www.eits.fr/courses/	Dry lab / wet lab	Offers 13 advanced courses in various fields
Core skills in laparoscopic surgery	Cuschieri Skills Centre, University of Dundee, United Kingdom	http://www.dundee.ac.uk/surgicalskills/courses/generalsurgery/coreskillsformerlykeyskillsinlaparoscopic/	Dry lab	
Intermediate skills for laparoscopic surgeons	Cuschieri Skills Centre, University of Dundee, United Kingdom	http://www.dundee.ac.uk/surgicalskills/courses/generalsurgery/intermediateskillsforlaparoscopicsurgeons/	Dry lab	

(*Continued*)

Table 3.3. Continued

Course name	Location	Webpage link	Type	Notes
Laparoscopic suturing	Cuschieri Skills Centre, University of Dundee, United Kingdom	http://www.dundee.ac.uk/surgicalskills/courses/generalsurgery/laparoscopicsuturingcourse/	Dry lab	
Cuschieri skills centre, other courses	Cuschieri Skills Centre, University of Dundee, United Kingdom	http://www.dundee.ac.uk/surgicalskills/courses/urology/	Dry lab	Simulator course in various fields including urology
Advanced laparoscopic surgery	AESCULAP Akademie, Berlin, Germany	http://www.aesculap-academy.com/		
Comprehensive urological laparoscopy	AESCULAP Akademie, Berlin, Germany	http://www.aesculap-academy.com/		
Advanced minimally invasive paediatric surgery	AESCULAP Akademie, Berlin, Germany	http://www.aesculap-academy.com/		
Minimal access surgery training	Birmingham Women's Hospital, MAST Unit, England	http://medweb.bham.ac.uk/mast/	Dry lab	

Danish Courses

Basal laparoskopi	Rigshospitalet, København	http://www.rigshospitalet.dk/menu/AFDELINGER/Juliane+Marie+Centret/Klinikker/Gynaekologisk+Klinik/Forskning/Simulatortraening/Kurset_Basal_Laparoskopi.htm	Simulator
U-kursus Urologisk laparoskopi	Århus Universitetshospital, Skejby, Århus	http://www.ydu.dk/index.php/kalender/event/2/82ojff47op5nivq6u0remdn87g	
Laparoskopi kurser i regi af MIUC	Minimal Invasiv Udviklings Center, Aalborg sygehus, Aalborg	http://www.miuc.dk/	
Kursusoversigt	MIUC	http://www.miuc.dk/index.php?menu_id=3	

Article describing different aspects of training in laparoscopy:
http://eu-acme.org/europeanurology/upload_articles/Training%20in%20Laparoscopy.pdf

Figure 3.1. Training scenario MIDC Module 1

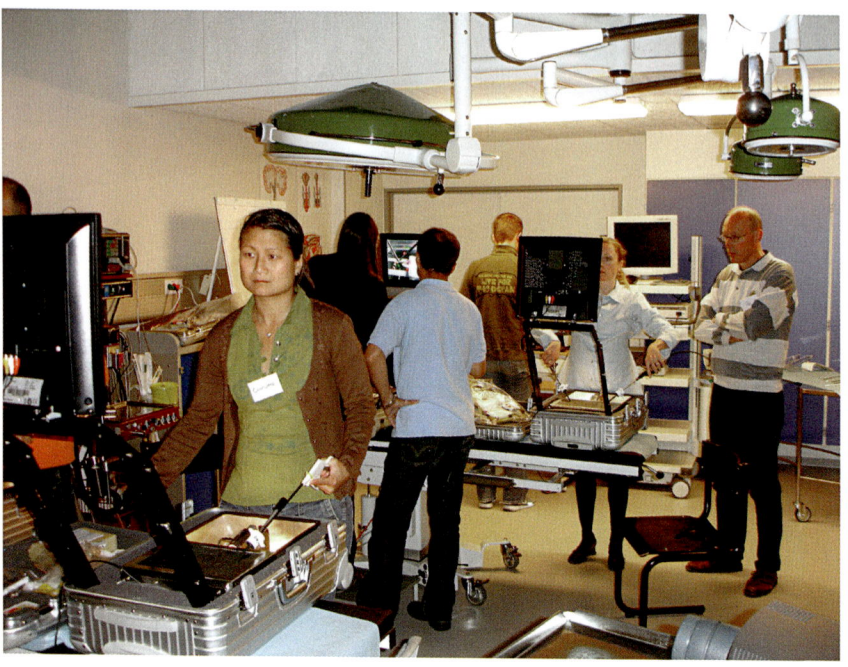

Figure 3.2. Training scenario MIDC Module 2

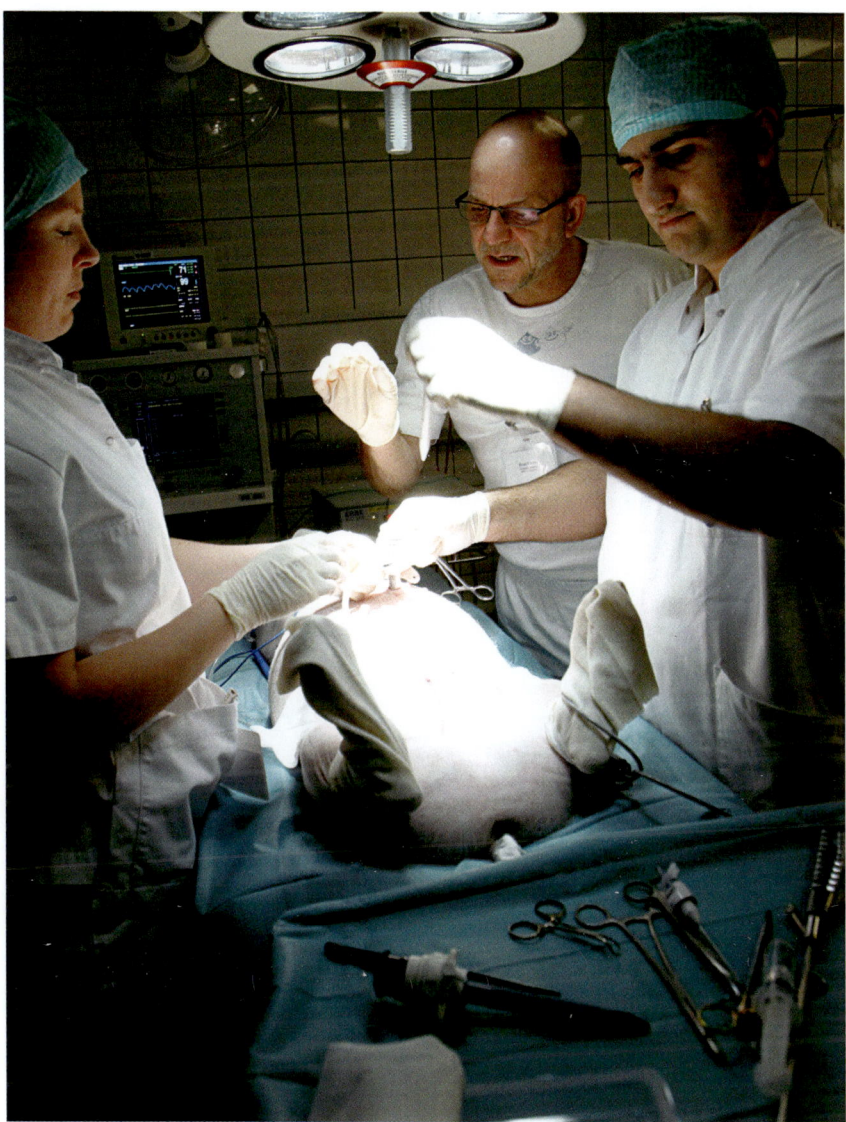

Figure 3.3. Training scenario MIDC Module 2

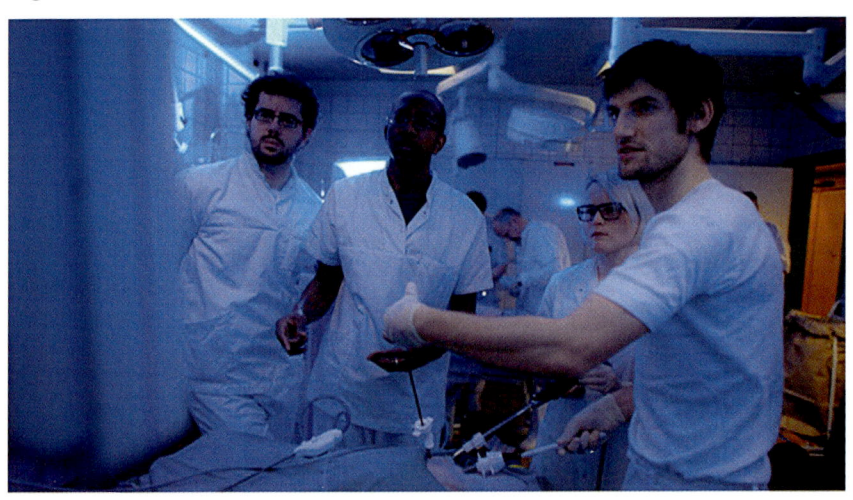

Figure 3.4. Training scenario MIDC Module 2

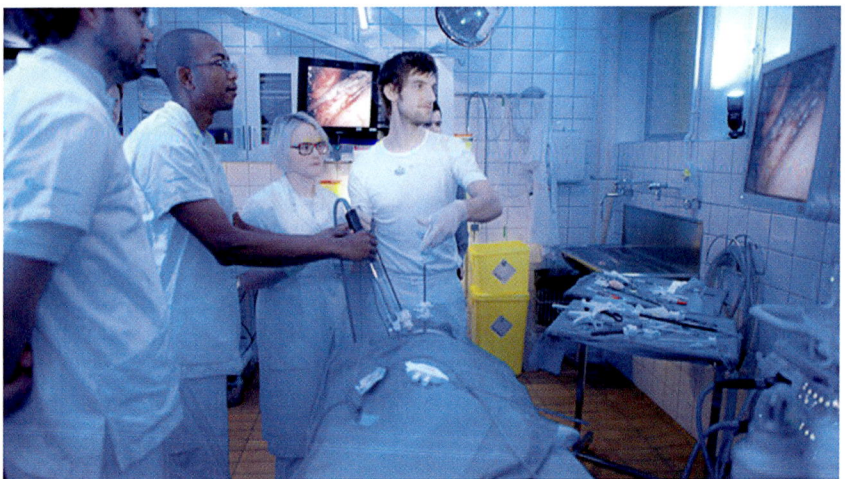

References

1. Gaba DM, DeAnda A. A comprehensive anesthesia simulation environment: re-creating the operating room for research and training. *Anesthesiology*. 1988;69:387–394.
2. Gordon JA, Brown DFM, Armstrong EG. Can a simulated critical care encounter accelerate basic science learning among preclinical medical students? A pilot study. *Simul Healthc*. 2006;1:13–17.
3. Marx T, Baldwin BR, Kittle CF. A cardiovascular simulator for the evaluation of prosthetic aortic valves. *J Thorac Cardiovasc Surg*. 1959;38:412–418.
4. Denson J, Abrahamson S. A computer-controlled patient simulator. *JAMA*. 1969;208:504–508.
5. Gaba DM, DeAnda A. A comprehensive anesthesia simulation environment: re-creating the operating room for research and training. *Anesthesiology*. 1988;69:387–394.
6. Shamim Khan M, Ahmed K, Gavazzi A, et al. Development and implementation of centralized simulation training: evaluation of feasibility, acceptability and construct validity. *BJU Int*. 2013;111:518–523.
7. Valero RJ, Moanack J, Cruz G, Sánchez-Ismayel A, Sánchez-Salas R, García-Seguí A. Animal model for training in laparoscopic pyeloplasty. *Actas Urol Esp*. 2012;36:54–59.
8. Zevin B, Aggarwal R, Grantcharov TP. Simulation-based training and learning curves in laparoscopic Roux-en-Y gastric bypass. *Br J Surg*. 2012;99:887–895.
9. Torricelli FC, Guglielmetti G, Duarte RJ, Srougi M. Laparoscopic skill laboratory in urological surgery: tools and methods for resident training. *Int Braz J Urol*. 2011;37:108–111.
10. Lund L, Høj L, Poulsen J, Funch P, Nilsson T. Organisation of basic training in laparoscopic surgery *Ugeskr læger*. 2010;172:436–440.
11. Lund L, Dubrowski A, Carnahan H. A modular approach for training laparoscopy to urologists. *BJU Int*. 2007;100:1216–1218.
12. Dunnington GL. The art of mentoring. *Am J Surg* 1996;171:604–607.
13. Bariol SV, Tolley DA. Training and mentoring in urology: the 'LAP' generation. *BJU Int*. 2004;93:913–914.
14. Matsuda T, Ono Y, Terachi T, et al. The endoscopic surgical skill qualification system in urological laparoscopy: a novel system in Japan. *J Urol*. 2006;176:2168–2172.
15. Davenport K, Timoney AG, Keeley FX, Joyce A, Downey P and members of the BAUS Section of Endourology. A three-year review of the British

Association of Urological Surgeons Section of Endourology Laparoscopic Nephrectomy Audit. *BJU Int.* 2006;97:333–337.
16. Grantcharov TP, Funch-Jensen P. Can everyone achieve proficiency with the laparoscopic technique? Learning curve patterns in technical skills acquisition. *Am J Surg.* 2009;197:447–449.
17. Aggarwal R, Tully A, Grantcharov T et al. Virtual reality simulation training can improve technical skills during laparoscopic salpingectomy for ectopic pregnancy. *BJOG.* 2006;113:1382–1387.
18. Gurusamy KS, Aggarwal R, Palanivelu L, et al. Virtual reality training for surgical trainees in laparoscopic surgery. *Cochrane Database Syst Rev.* 2009;1:CD006575.

Chapter 4

FULL PROCEDURAL SURGICAL SIMULATION

Laura Nicol and Irfan Ahmed

Introduction

Almost half a century ago, the invention of Resusci Anne (Figure 4.1) in 1960 was the first example of a tool for practising a full procedural simulation, but it is only in the past decade that full procedural simulation has rapidly evolved into a useful learning tool for both trainees and experienced doctors. Full procedural simulation refers to the technique of imitating a full operation and, as such, has a number of separate components. The components of a procedure are different from the simple rehearsal of a skill as they take into account both technical and non-technical skills, allowing them to be integrated simultaneously. The invention and validation of distributed simulation has shown how high-fidelity simulators can be made available to wider audiences, improving access to simulation education for all (1).

This shift in paradigm of learning has been brought about by a number of factors. Firstly, in surgery the traditional apprenticeship model is no longer sufficient to develop trainees' skills, as many operations which they historically used as learning cases are no longer performed due to the introduction of minimally invasive techniques and use of video technology via endoscopes and operating microscopes. This has removed many educational opportunities for trainees, leading to a lack of basic procedural operating skills. More universally, the reduction in training hours due to initiatives such as the European Working Time Directive (EWTD) has led to a shortening of the time available for trainees to acquire a full complement of surgical skills (1). Finally, initiatives in patient safety stemming from investigations and recommendations such as those of the Bristol Inquiry (1998) have forced surgeons to come to think of surgical training as the swift acquisition of necessary technical skills in a safe environment that poses no threat to patients (2).

As our technology and operative equipment becomes more controlled and precise, students move away from practising tying knots around chair legs in operating theatres and look for more sophisticated tools to hone their skills quickly and thoroughly. The old surgical teaching method of 'see one, do one, teach one' must now be firmly consigned to the dustbin of history.

The transfer of skills from simulation environments such as virtual reality (VR) to the operating room (OR) should be sequential and controlled. The healthcare industry should follow the models adopted by the airline industry. The transfer of skills from VR to OR was first described in 1993 by Satava, based on an aviation model (5). He claimed that, 'The surgical resident of the future will learn new perspectives on surgical anatomy and repeatedly practise surgical procedures until they are perfect before performing surgery on patients'. In the findings of the Bristol Inquiry, the response by the senate stated that, 'there should be no learning curve as far as patient safety is concerned' (6). The sequential progression of skills from VR to the dry lab, then from the wet lab (including animal models) to a live procedure performed under mentorship, should enable the development of transferrable skills which can be used in the final stage of surgical training: performing a safe procedure independently.

Several studies have shown that VR training has clear benefits that can be transferred to the operating theatre. Trainees who practise skills using a VR system consistently operate faster and with fewer errors than those who learn only from an apprenticeship model, i.e., moving from observing to assisting and, finally, performing. One such study by Seymour et al. compared surgical residents assigned to a standard training group to those adopting both standard and VR training (using the MIST-VR system) in the performance of a laparoscopic cholecystectomy under the supervision of senior surgeons (7). They demonstrated that the VR-trained group took 29% less time than the standard training group and made five times fewer errors. Following on from this study, Ahlberg et al. showed similar results in their research (Figure 4.2) (4). It is clear from these studies that the development of skills with the use of procedural simulation is both swift and safe.

Although such studies provide arguments for the use of procedural simulation, the concept of frequently evaluating outcomes will remain vital to future assessments of the benefits of simulation. More data is required before it will become routine, as no matter how innovative and highly evolved our simulators, if we cannot demonstrate their benefits to trainees in the operating room, they are rendered useless.

This chapter aims to give an overview of full procedural simulation, incorporating virtual operating theatres and distributed simulation. It will define the components of simulation and highlight the validation of its effectiveness in terms of content validation, construct validation, feasibility, acceptability and educational impact.

The Virtual or Mission Rehearsal

Although errors can be reduced using simulation, even the most advanced simulation tools such as the LapSim cholecystectomy (Figure 4.4), a state of the art laparoscopic cholecystectomy simulator, can only allow trainees to target a specific skills area. Studies have shown that errors in the operating room are more often due to problems with surgeons' non-technical skills, i.e., communication, teamwork, decision making, situational awareness, task management and leadership, rather than their technical ability to perform a procedure. As the current simulators only address technical skills, other components, including non-technical skills, must be integrated into the process to ensure the safe completion of any whole procedure. This is what is termed 'mission rehearsal' in literature, and already has an established place in the military and aviation (2).

Based on this idea, a recent conception within medical education is the creation of a virtual operating room (VOR). This concept is vital if simulation is to be used as a tool for training within an established curriculum. New integrated simulation systems can now enable full procedural simulation for various complete surgical procedures, such as the VIST system for endovascular surgery (Figure 4.5). VORs will be essential for any training programme as they combine teaching with an assessment of non-technical as well as technical skills, an idea already demonstrated in a 2007 pilot feasibility study (2).

Paige et al. formed a simulation-based interdisciplinary team-training programme for the operating room (8). They created a VOR (Figure 4.6) and a three-hour scenario involving a laparoscopic cholecystectomy with an intraoperative cardiac arrhythmia, which the team had to diagnose properly and treat promptly to stop the patient developing cardiac arrest. In this way, the scenario involved teamwork and many of the behavioural competencies associated with highly effective teams.

We feel that mission rehearsal in surgery is possible with current technology. Skills can be transferred and the techniques demonstrated correlate well with a live patient procedure. There is no better development for the technical and non-technical skills of a surgical resident than to train in a similar environment to that they will be exposed to in the future. As we all know, practice makes perfect.

Distributed Simulation

Widespread uptake of simulators is limited by several factors, such as cost, time, storage and fair access for all trainees. The idea of a mobile surgical simulation unit aims to reduce the cost of investing in simulators, as well as the issue of storage. It also ensures that all trainees, regardless of how remote their location, receive equal access to this training resource.

Many innovative mobile simulation systems are being piloted worldwide. One such system has been introduced in the Republic of Ireland (3). This portable simulation unit visits each hospital for one day every six weeks. Over their two-year core training programme, the trainees cover technical skills such as knot tying, leading up to the performance of full surgical procedures. This allows over 200 trainees equal access to resources to learn surgical techniques and procedures which are taught to them in their own hospitals by their consultant supervisors. Although this system is set up for junior surgeons, higher surgical residents can also benefit by attending the sessions in teaching simulation to learn new and more advanced techniques.

More recently, a mobile simulation unit has been piloted at Imperial College, London (3). This portable simulated theatre environment uses an inflatable 360-degree 'igloo' to provide a self-contained environment which screens trainees from the outside world and, therefore, perpetuates their suspension of disbelief. This 'distributed simulation environment' has been shown to have strong face and content validity when compared with a laparoscopic box trainer. This has a number of implications for simulation training, as the authors have demonstrated that high-fidelity full procedural simulation can be achieved in a low-cost environment which makes it a useful tool for teaching in remote and rural settings which cover large geographical areas.

Evidence for Validation

Being able to measure validity is an important part of any innovation or new process. Before we can use simulation as a tool to help trainees improve and to then assess those skills, we have to be able to show that it is a reliable resource which will teach trainee operations as well as or better than operating on live patients. As with any new system, validation is essential before it can be added to an educational curriculum.

Various components of validity need to be considered in this process. Face validity is the extent to which the simulation resembles a real-life situation. Construct validity, on the other hand, is the degree to which the concept or theory matches the outcome, i.e., whether simulation produces improved outcomes in terms of surgical skills acquisition: a test has shown construct validity if it is able to distinguish between different levels of experience in the operators. Concurrent validity compares the test to the gold standard, assessing whether the simulation trains students as well as practice on a live patient would. Similarly, predictive validity determines whether the student's performance on a simulator corresponds to actual performance in the operating room.

To this end, a limited number of studies have been undertaken to demonstrate validity. The concept of construct validity pertaining to simulation was established as early as 2003 in a study comparing expert and novice surgeons on a VR laparoscopic cholecystectomy simulator (3). This study compared 'experts' (defined as surgeons having performed over 100 laparoscopic cholecystectomies) and 'novice' surgeons, who had no experience in this operation at all. The results showed that the experts were significantly faster to complete all three attempts, but there was also an increase in the score over the three operations in both groups. Having demonstrated an improved outcome in terms of skills acquisition, therefore, the construct is valid.

Face and construct validity have also been determined in later studies using VR training for robotic surgery (9). Participants were asked to perform a 'ring transfer' task (Figure 4.7). In this task, the expert surgeons performed better than the novices on total task time, economy of movement and time spent outside the centre of the platform's workspace. All surgeons found the VR simulator to be acceptable, and thus the study proves both face and construct validity.

There are very few studies looking at concurrent validity, presumably due to the difficulties in developing and conducting such a study. There have been several small-scale attempts to establish concurrent validity, such a 2009 study which aimed to determine whether the trainees' performance in the operating theatre correlated to their performance on a VR laparoscopic trainer (10). Performance was assessed using a modified Objective Structured Assessment of Technical Skill (OSATS). Participants performed seven basic skills repeated three times. They then went on to perform one laparoscopic cholecystectomy on a live patient that was recorded and assessed by two observers on various parameters, such as time used, error score and economy of movement, which were also used by the simulation unit to score the participants. Correlations were drawn between operative performance (assessed by two observers) and performance in the virtual environment (assessed by the computer), which concluded that the simulator was comparative to the gold standard and therefore demonstrates concurrent validity.

Developing and maintaining a high-specification VR environment is not without cost and even a simple VR simulator involves a significant investment of both time and money. Such investments in the fields of aviation and the military has led to the invention of cutting-edge technology. The issue of purchasing simulators within the wider budget for surgical education remains topical and it is unclear who will be responsible for this investment. Although at present both distributed simulation units and fixed simulators are used for the acquisition of basic skills, with the right investment, more high-fidelity simulators could be developed to teach the senior trainees very specific procedures. The validity and reliability of simulation needs to be assessed rigorously in order to prove the benefits to both the trainee and the patient before such an investment is likely.

Conclusions

Simulation has existed in the fields of aviation and in the military for many years. It was originally developed to give pilots and soldiers the opportunity to practise high-risk manoeuvres, honing their skills in a controlled environment before using them in real life situations.

Medical simulation systems are available which allow the trainees to practise full procedural simulation in various situations, improving patient safety. This has now been shown to serve as a valid training tool that can significantly improve trainees' performance in the operating room. Simulation will improve patient safety by reducing the learning curve, moving training away from patients to a low-risk environment.

We strongly believe that the introduction of full procedural simulation in the medical curriculum will enhance the delivery of the safe transfer of technical and non-technical skills to medical professionals.

Figures and Tables

Figure 4.1. The resuscitation department at the centre for health science, Raigmore Hospital, Inverness

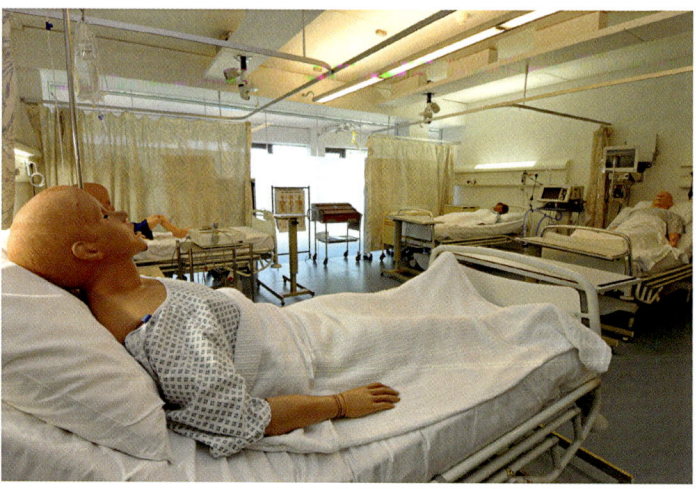

Resusci Anne manikins, now widely used in medical schools, were based on the death mask of 'L'Inconnue de la Seine', a young unidentified woman whose body was pulled from the River Seine in the late 1880s. Picture taken by facilitators at the centre for health science.

Figure 4.2. Frequency of each error type during exposure of Calot's triangle

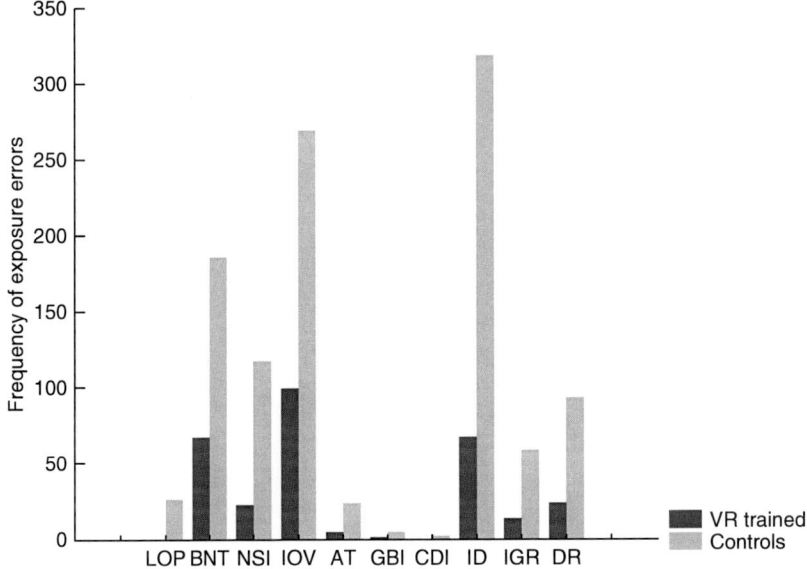

LOP, lack of progress; BNT, burn non-target tissue; NSI, non-target structure injury; IOV, instrument out of view; AT, attending take over; GBI, gallbladder injury; CDI, cystic duct injury; ID, inappropriate dissection; IGR, incorrect angle of gallbladder retraction; DR, dropped retraction. Permission obtained from Elsevier (4).

Figure 4.3. Frequency of error for each error type during gallbladder dissection

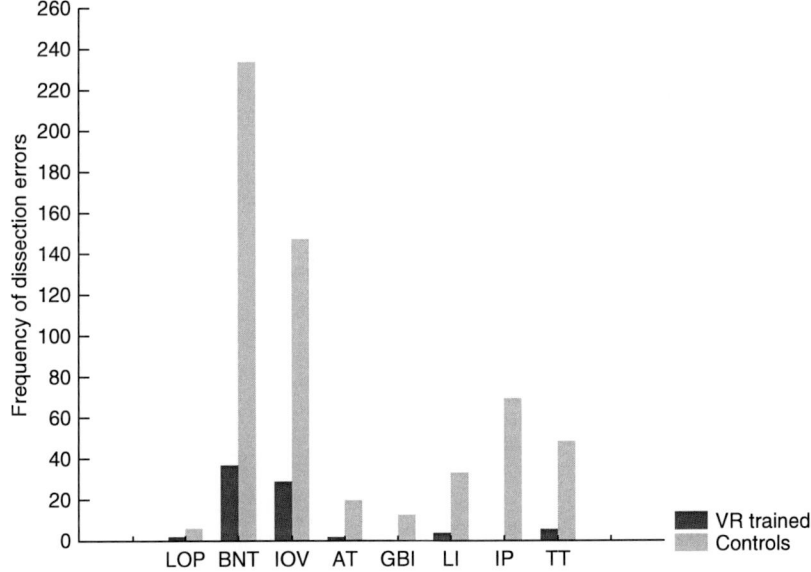

LOP, lack of progress; BNT, burn non-target; IOV, instrument out of view; AT, attending take over; GBI, gallbladder injury; LI, liver injury; IP, incorrect plane of dissection; TT, tearing tissue. Permission obtained from Elsevier (4).

Figure 4.4. The LapSim cholecystectomy simulates the critical steps in a laparoscopic cholecystectomy

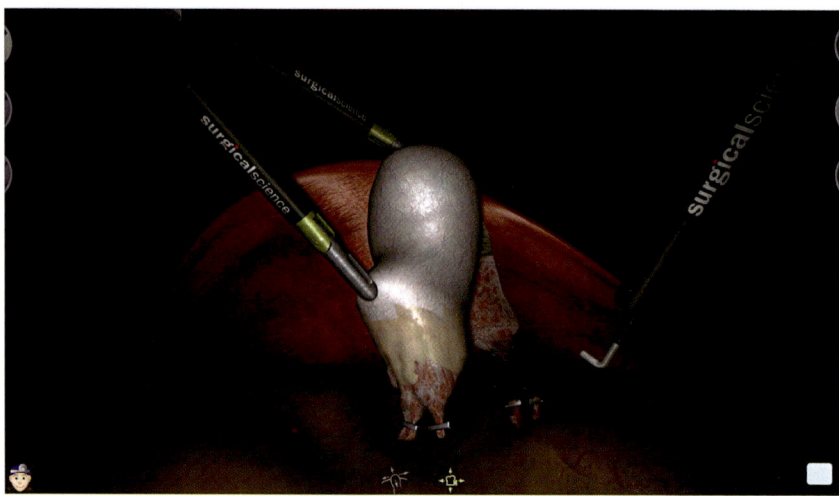

In the first part, the cystic duct and artery are clipped and cut off. In the second part, the gallbladder is separated and removed from the liver. Image supplied by Surgical Science.

Figure 4.5. The VIST system, a high-fidelity endovascular simulator

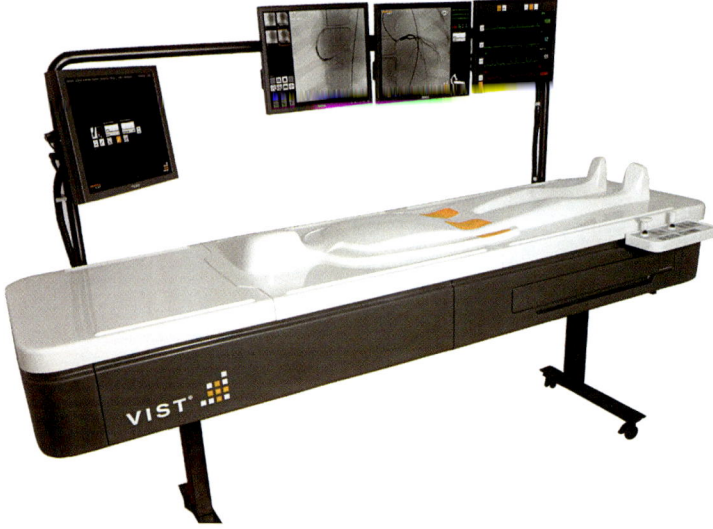

Photo provided by Mentice AB, Gothenburg, Sweden.

Figure 4.6. The VOR for endovascular training

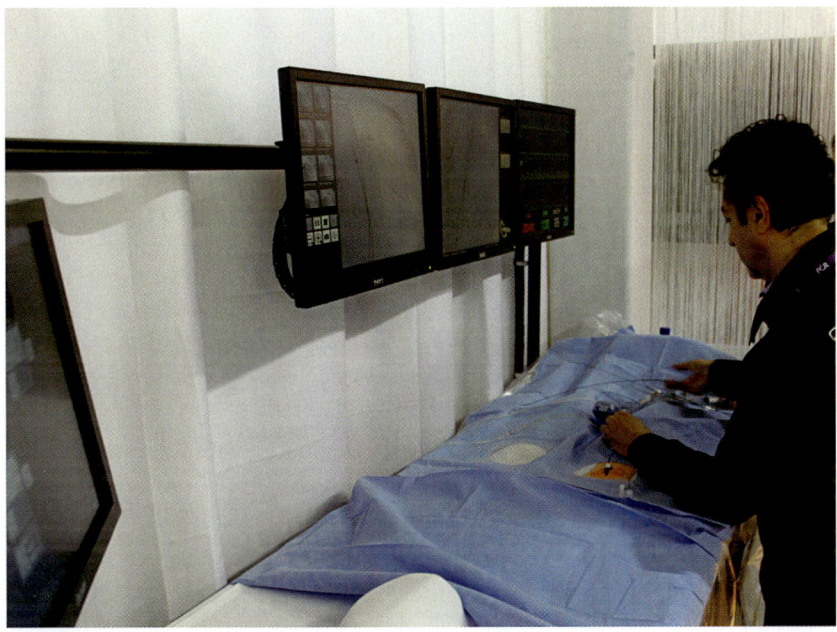

Photo provided by Mentice AB, Gothenburg, Sweden.

Figure 4.7. A simple ring transfer task in which the operator must pick up the pink ring and place it over the highlighted peg

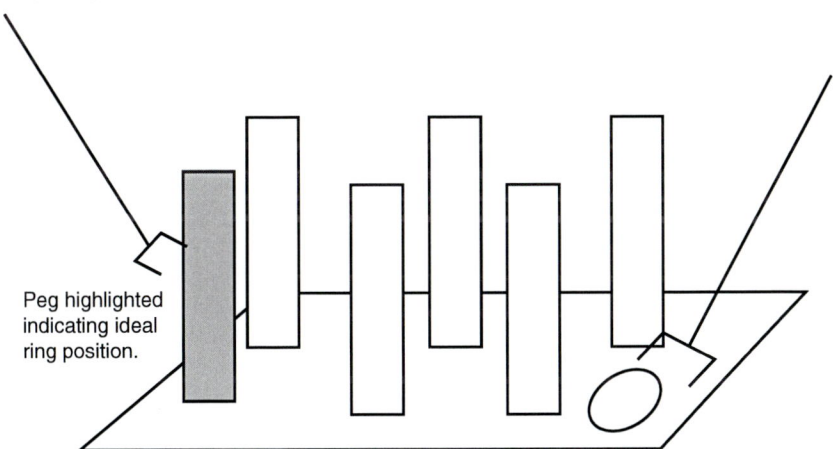

References

1. Association of Surgeons of Great Britain and Ireland. *The Impact of EWTD on Delivery of Surgical Services: A Consensus Statement.* ASGBI; 2008.
2. Carter FJ, Schijven MP, Aggarwal R, et al. Consensus guidelines for validation of virtual reality surgical simulators. *Simul Healthc.* 2006;1:171.
3. Schijven M, Jakimowicz J. Construct validity: experts and novices performing on the Xitact LS500 laparoscopy simulator. *Surg Endosc.* 2003;17:803–810.
4. Ahlberg G, Enochsson L, Gallagher AG, et al. Proficiency-based VR training significantly reduces the error rate for residents during their first ten laparoscopic cholecystectomies. *Am J Surg.* 2007;193:797–804.
5. Satava RM. Virtual reality surgical simulator: the first steps. *Surg Endosc.* 1993;7(3):203–205.
6. Bristol Royal Infirmary Inquiry (2001). The inquiry into the management of care of children receiving complex heart surgery at the Bristol Royal Infirmary. http://www.bristol-inquiry.org.uk/. Accessed 11th April 2012.
7. Seymour N, Gallagher A, Roman S, O'Brien M, Bansal V, Andersen D, Satava R. Virtual reality training improves operating room performance: results of a randomized, double-blinded study. *Ann Surg.* 2002;236(4): 458–464.
8. Paige J, Kozmenko V, Morgan B, Howell DS, Chauvin S, Hilton C, Cohn I Jr, O'Leary JP. From the flight deck to the operating room: an initial pilot study of the feasibility and potential impact of true interdisciplinary team training using high-fidelity simulation. *J Surg Educ.* 2007;64(6): 369–377.
9. Lendvay T, Casale P, Sweet R, Peters C. Initial validation of a virtual-reality robotic simulator. *J Robot Surg.* 2008;2(3):145–149.
10. Kundhal PS, Grantcharov TP. Psychomotor performance measured in a virtual environment correlates with technical skills in the operating room. *Surg Endosc.* 2009;23(3):645–649.

Chapter 5

DEVELOPING NON-TECHNICAL SKILLS

James Brewin and Peter Jaye

Introduction

Surgery, perhaps more than any other branch of medicine, has been defined by the technical skills of its clinicians, and this has meant that the acquisition of these skills has taken primacy over other training requirements. However, the practice of surgery contains far more than high-quality technical skills. These other skills are termed non-technical skills (NTS) and include cognitive and social skills such as decision making, situation awareness, professionalism, teamwork and communication.

There is increasing evidence that deficiencies in NTS exist in surgical teams and that this can significantly affect team performance and patient safety. Clearly current models of surgical training do not adequately ensure the development of these skills and healthcare still 'lags unacceptably behind other safety-critical industries such as aviation' (House of Commons Health Committee, 2009).

These NTS are not innate personality traits but can be taught and developed through training. Several authors and government bodies have called for improved training to address this skills gap and simulation has emerged as a powerful training tool to help achieve this (1, 2).

This chapter will first discuss the importance of NTS in healthcare and assuring patient safety and also highlight deficiencies of NTS in surgical practice. Secondly, training methods to improve NTS will be discussed with an emphasis on high-fidelity simulation-based training, which is being increasingly used as a tool to develop and assess these skills in healthcare. Finally, we will discuss how NTS training can be integrated into the surgical curriculum in order to improve team performance and patient safety.

The Importance of Non-technical Skills

NTS are the 'cognitive and social skills that complement workers' technical skills' and include abilities such as decision making, situational awareness, communication and teamwork (3). The importance of NTS in high-risk industries was initially recognised in aviation following the analysis of several high-profile disasters such as the Tenerife airport disaster in 1977. Root cause analysis of errors in aviation as well as other high-risk industries (e.g., military, nuclear, petrochemical) has shown that deficiencies in NTS cause or contribute to 80% of errors (3). These industries have recognised the importance of NTS in team performance and embraced NTS training (4, 5).

In comparison to other safety-critical industries, healthcare has been slow to appreciate the importance of NTS. Several high-profile medical errors have been caused by deficiencies in NTS and, partly in response to these cases, the healthcare industry is starting to appreciate the importance of NTS for patient safety (see Table 5.1). There is now a significant body of evidence which demonstrates that the quality of a healthcare professional's NTS has a significant impact on patient safety.

The importance of NTS applies to the operating room (OR) perhaps more than it does to any other clinical environment. The OR is a complex, high-risk environment where a team of professionals must work together to optimise patient outcome. Training has traditionally focused on technical skills but performance is also dependant on systems factors and NTS (see Figure 1).

Errors occur in any system, but in surgery at least 15% of patients experience an adverse event and up to half of these are preventable; this would be unacceptable in other high-reliability organisations (6). Several studies have identified poor communication, teamwork and decision making in surgical teams and it is these errors in NTS that cause the majority of errors in the OR (6, 7). Furthermore, deficiencies in NTS are associated with poor technical performance of the operating surgeon and higher post-operative morbidity and mortality (8, 9). Unfortunately these deficiencies are compounded by poor insight as the majority of surgeons cannot accurately judge their own NTS (10). In addition, team members often have differences in opinion about each other's NTS performance and team members do not always appreciate the importance of NTS on performance (11, 12).

Non-technical Skills for Surgery

NTS can be classified into cognitive (e.g., decision making, situational awareness, planning), social (e.g., communication, teamwork, leadership) and personal resource factors (e.g., ability to cope with stress or fatigue) (3). The behavioural markers that reflect NTS cannot be assumed to be the same in different work environments, therefore several studies have been conducted to identify behaviours that reflect NTS performance in the OR (13). Scoring systems to assess these skills have also been developed.

One of the most thoroughly validated scoring systems is the Non-technical Skills for Surgeons rating system (NOTSS) which was developed by the Industrial Psychology Research Centre at the University of Aberdeen (www.abdn.ac.uk/iprc/notss) (14, 15). The non-technical skills (NOTECHS) scale, originally developed for aviation, has also been adapted and validated for use in the OR (16). Although these scoring systems are slightly different, the underlying research has identified several NTS domains that are important for optimal performance in the OR. Observable behaviours related to these NTS have also been identified so that these skills can be objectively rated (see Table 5.2).

These scoring systems have helped to identify key NTS for the OR and provide a framework to describe these skills to surgeons. They have been predominantly used for research but can also be used to assess the effects of educational programmes on NTS performance. They also have the potential to act as structured feedback tools for training in both simulated- and work-based settings and have been successfully used across various training programmes.

The above studies have highlighted deficiencies in the NTS of surgical teams and provided a framework of NTS in the OR. Fortunately NTS are not innate personality traits but are skills that can be taught and improved. Lessons from other industries have shown that training can improve NTS in the workplace. Although the research in healthcare is less developed there is increasing evidence to support the value of NTS training. Several strategies have been used to improve NTS in the workplace but in healthcare, as in other industries, simulation-based team training has emerged as one of the best ways to achieve this (3, 17, 18).

Human Patient Simulation as a Training Tool for NTS

Some of the most widely used techniques for NTS training have developed from crew resource management (CRM) in aviation, which uses a mixture of didactic teaching, workshops and simulated scenarios. The aim of CRM training is to provide participants with the skills to prevent errors or, when errors do occur, to mitigate the effects of these errors (3). Several industries including healthcare have developed and adapted this model. One of the first medical specialities to utilise this model was anaesthetics with the development of crisis resource management training pioneered by David Gaba and colleagues in the 1990s (19). Crisis resource management training includes lectures and workshops but there is a heavy emphasis on team-based simulation training using high-fidelity patient simulators.

Human patient simulation (HPS) utilises life-sized manikins placed in simulated or real clinical environments. Simulated clinical scenarios are developed to practise skills in realistic team-based environments, often incorporating a simulated crisis. This is followed by a detailed debriefing session which is used to analyse the performance and identify NTS and behaviours that if applied to the workplace can improve performance. These high-fidelity training scenarios are probably most useful when implemented as part of multidisciplinary team training with all members of the team (20, 21).

These training principles have been successfully applied to training the OR team. Several groups have combined a realistic OR environment with a high-fidelity human patient manikin and part-task surgical trainers. The manikin can reproduce realistic patient physiology while the part-task surgical simulator can recreate a technical aspect of a surgical procedure. The aim is to create an environment with enough realism for participants to suspend disbelief and display realistic team behaviours which can be discussed and analysed during subsequent debriefings. This type of training has been used in simulated OR environments as well as for in-situ training where simulators are used in the real OR (22–24, 25). Fully simulated settings have the advantage that they can be conducted in simulation centres and are available whatever the clinical pressures. They also have integrated audiovisual recording equipment allowing playback of the scenario during the debriefing process. In-situ simulation training has the advantage of being able to test systems factors whilst teaching NTS to 'organic' teams actually present in the real environment. However it may be difficult to organise in a busy OR environment, and dedicated teaching facilities and audiovisual equipment may not be available to help deliver an effective debriefing.

In order to implement effective simulation-based training, scenarios must be carefully developed and piloted in an effort to deliver specific learning objectives and ensure adequate levels of realism. Furthermore, with inter- and multi-professional team training the scenarios must satisfy the learning needs of a variety of professionals: it is essential that the inter- and multi-professional faculty develop and deliver the scenarios.

Although scenario design is vitally important in order to allow participants to suspend disbelief, the post-scenario debriefing has consistently been identified as the most important aspect of the learning experience (21, 26). In fact, without debriefing sessions NTS may not improve at all with simulation training (21, 26). A typical debriefing process involves analysing the simulated performance, often with the help of video playback. It is not only the candidates participating in the scenario who can benefit from each scenario. All the other candidates on the course watch each scenario and should be encouraged to actively participate in the debriefing process. This should give all candidates the opportunity to discuss the scenario and the relevant NTS and learn throughout the course.

In order to enhance adult learning and encourage positive behavioural change a facilitative rather than an instructional approach appears to be superior (3, 26). This approach allows learners to actively participate in the post-scenario debrief with a skilled facilitator who guides the process. The facilitator can provide feedback, encourage learners to analyse specific behaviours and NTS, create a safe learning environment and help learners to apply their knowledge to work-based settings. In our experience a structured debrief approach is essential. This model deals with technical skills before moving on to NTS and may be particularly important in surgery where technical skills acquisition and practice has traditionally defined clinical practice.

The presence of a trained and experienced facilitator is vitally important to optimise learning during these debriefing sessions (3, 26). Consequently, several institutions offer training for simulation-based educators to help improve debriefing skills and learn how to utilise the validated NTS scoring systems (e.g., NOTSS and NOTECHS). Support by senior faculty, with or without the use of formal assessment tools, can help maintain and develop the teaching skills required to conduct an effective debriefing session.

Implementation of High-Fidelity Team-Based Simulation Training

As with any educational intervention, a needs assessment is usually the first step. As can be seen from the above studies on NTS in surgery, there is generally a need to improve NTS. Furthermore, rating scales such as NOTTS and NOTECHS can help identify specific deficiencies. In order to develop a simulation training programme, the 'five Ps' need to be established: *place* (adequate facilities, often a simulation facility), *products* (such as a high-fidelity manikin and part-task trainers), *pounds* (adequate funding), *positioning* (within the training curriculum) and *people* (27).

Positioning and people are particularly important. Ideally NTS training should be positioned appropriately in a spiral curriculum that is integrated into the training and professional development throughout a surgeon's career. Training programmes are able to focus on NTS that are particularly relevant to a practitioner at a given time (e.g., leadership training for senior clinicians). In our experience we have found that a partnership between surgical specialists and an experienced simulation faculty provides the most effective programme. The simulation faculty can help with curriculum development, teacher training and ensuring good quality facilitation of the debriefing sessions. Experienced simulation faculty can often be found in other specialities that have developed NTS training programmes such as anaesthetics and emergency medicine.

Evidence for Team-Based High-Fidelity Simulation in Surgery

Although human patient simulation-based team training is generally accepted as the best way to improve NTS and enhance patient safety, the evidence base is still developing. Kirkpatrick described four levels of evaluation for educational interventions:

> Level 1 – did the students enjoy the experience?
> Level 2 – is there evidence of learning?
> Level 3 – is there evidence of behavioural change?
> Level 4 – is there evidence of better outcomes? (28)

Several studies in surgery have shown that team-based high-fidelity OR simulation fulfils Kirkpatrick Levels 1 to 3. Training is well received and has been shown to improve team performance and NTS in the simulated setting (24, 22, 29). However it is very difficult to establish whether training definitely improves patient safety (Kirkpatrick Level 4). Even in the airline industry, where there is significant evidence that CRM training improves team performance, there is no convincing Kirkpatrick Level 4 evidence that it improves safety (5). However this has not prevented the widespread adoption of simulation-based training focused on NTS. As David Gaba states:

> No industry in which human lives depend on the skilled performance of responsible operators has waited for unequivocal proof of the benefits of simulation before embracing it. Why should healthcare be any different? (30)

Available evidence shows that simulation-based training improves performance, and this should encourage continuing efforts to train surgeons in NTS. However we should continue to try to evaluate the effects of these training programmes on patient outcome.

Other Strategies to Improve NTS

High-fidelity simulation-based training is not the only way to develop NTS and several other training approaches have been used. Furthermore, non-training interventions such as the introduction of the pre-operative checklist can improve NTS in the OR and improve patient outcomes (31).

Examples of other training methods aimed at improving team performance and NTS include computer- or paper-based simulations to aid decision making, cross-training to improve role awareness, assertiveness training to improve communication and team coordination training (3).

Novel training programmes to improve NTS are also being developed and applied to surgery. An example of this is the randomised controlled trial by Wetzel et al., who found that stress management training not only reduced stress during a simulated OR crisis but also improved NTS (32). Novel training programmes such as these can add to the array of training tools available to improve performance in the OR.

Although the majority of literature has focused on NTS training in formal learning environments such as the simulation centre or the classroom, there is no reason why NTS cannot be developed in the workplace. Debriefing can be performed after routine or critical workplace events, and scoring systems such as NOTSS can be used to focus on and analyse NTS.

This chapter has focused on simulation as a training tool, partly because it is one of the most widely used techniques for developing NTS. However, the choice of training method will depend on training needs and available recourses. Further research is needed to establish how and when these different training methods can be used to optimise team performance and how best to integrate these training methods into healthcare curricula. Combinations of qualitative and quantitative research methodologies are probably needed if we are to understand the complexities of using these educational strategies to improve team performance.

The Future of Simulation-Based Training for NTS

Training of surgeons in NTS is still in its infancy, but with increasing recognition of the importance of NTS, particularly in the OR, this is changing and several institutions now offer training programmes. As in other high-risk industries, simulation-based team training appears to be a powerful tool for teaching NTS but it is yet to be integrated into curricula in many countries.

In aviation NTS are taught using a three-phase model (3). Firstly, participants are introduced to NTS in a classroom-based course (the awareness phase). They then undergo numerous simulation-based exercises with detailed debriefing (practice phase) and finally they undergo continual intermittent training to maintain their skills. The reality in healthcare is that, although simulation-based training is used, we are still at the awareness phase. Hopefully the surgical curriculum will begin to formally include NTS training and with increasing training facilities and further research into NTS training there will be improvements in team performance and patient safety.

Conclusion

It is clear that the surgeon is not just 'a pair of hands' and that team performance is not dependant only on technical skills and knowlege. NTS have been shown to affect performance and patient outcomes in healthcare and, more specifically, in the complex, high-risk environment of the OR. Failures in these NTS have been demonstrated in surgery and there is an increasing recognition that formal training is needed to improve these skills. Despite this, training still focuses on technical skills and NTS have been learned in a much more ad hoc way such as by modelling the behaviours of respected seniors.

Surgery is starting to develop formal training models to improve and assess these skills. Although several training models can be used to develop NTS, high-fidelity simulation-based team training seems to be the most effective and it has been shown to improve performance when judged by validated rating scales. Surgical training is starting to include NTS, but with continuing developments and increasing simulation training capacity there is hope that NTS training can be fully integrated into the surgical curriculum.

Key Messages

1. NTS are vital in healthcare delivery and patient safety.
2. NTS have been shown to affect surgical performance and patient outcomes.
3. NTS are skills: they can be learned.
4. Simulation is an excellent tool for developing NTS.
5. For simulation to be effective it must be implemented well and high-quality debriefing skills are essential.

Figures and Tables

Table 5.1. High-profile medical errors in the United Kingdom which have highlighted deficiencies in NTS

Speciality	Critical incident	Failures in NTS
Urology (2000)	Graham Reeves – wrong site nephrectomy	Communication, situational awareness
Oncology (2001)	Wayne Jowett – intrathecal vincristine given in error	Situational awareness, communication, system errors
Anaesthetics/ ENT (2006)	Elaine Bromerly – failure to manage a can't intubate/can't ventilate scenario	Situational awareness, leadership, communication

Figure 5.1. Factors contributing to performance in the workplace

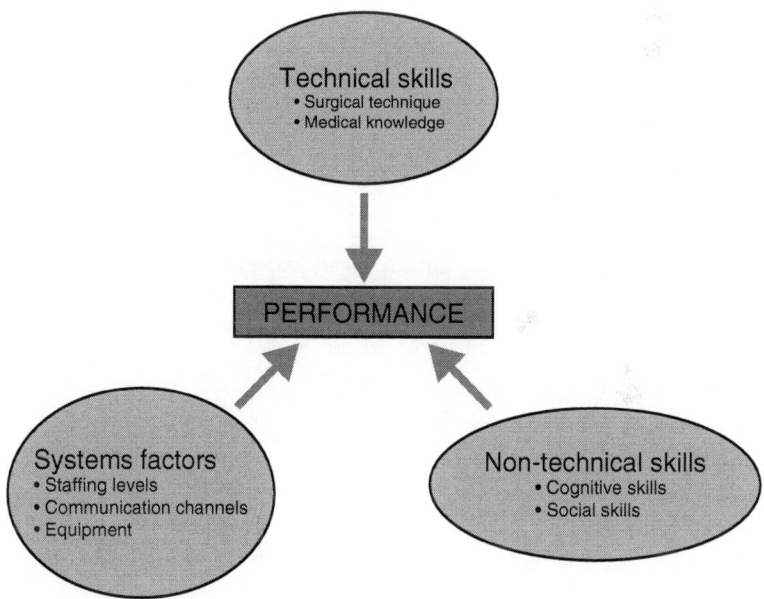

Table 5.2. Examples of components of NTS for the OR

Non-Technical Skill	Description	Examples of Good Behaviours
Communication (social skill)	Ability to clearly deliver and receive information	Clear and concise instructions Waits for check back
Teamwork (social skill)	Coordination of activities to optimise performance.	Supportive of other team members Values and utilises contributions of other team members
Leadership (social skill)	Ability of the team leader to optimise team performance	Does not permit corner cutting Utilisation of resources Manages time well
Situational awareness (cognitive skill)	Ability of the individual or team to accurately perceive the environment	Continuous monitoring of patient parameters Verbalises what is needed in the future
Decision making (cognitive skill)	The process of reaching a judgement or deciding on a course of action	Verbalises problem Communicates and implements decision Reviews/monitors outcome

Adapted from 3, 14, 16.

References

1. Youngson GG, Flin R. Patient safety in surgery: non-technical aspects of safe surgical performance. *Patient Saf Surg.* 2010;4(1):4.
2. CMO Annual Report. Safer medical practice: machines, manikins and polo mints. 2008. www.bmsc.co.uk/pdf/DH-096227.pdf. Accessed 12 December 2013.
3. Flin R, O'Connor P, Crichton M. *Safety at the Sharp End: A Guide to Non-Technical Skills.* Farnham: Ashgate; 2008.
4. Salas E, Burke CS, Bowers CA, Wilson KA. Team training in the skies: does crew resource management (CRM) training work? *Hum Factors.* 2001;43(4):641–674.
5. Salas E, Wilson KA, Burke CS, Wightman DC. Does crew resource management training work? An update, an extension, and some critical needs. *Hum Factors.* 2006;48(2):392–412.
6. Gawande AA, Zinner MJ, Studdert DM, Brennan TA. Analysis of errors reported by surgeons at three teaching hospitals. *Surgery.* 2003;133(6):614–621.

7. Rogers SO, Jr, Gawande AA, Kwaan M, et al. Analysis of surgical errors in closed malpractice claims at four liability insurers. *Surgery.* 2006;140(1):25–33.
8. Hull L, Arora S, Aggarwal R, Darzi A, Vincent C, Sevdalis N. The impact of non-technical skills on technical performance in surgery: a systematic review. *J Am Coll Surg.* 2012;214(2):214–230.
9. Mazzocco K, Petitti DB, Fong KT, et al. Surgical team behaviors and patient outcomes. *Am J Surg.* 2009;197(5):678–685.
10. Arora S, Miskovic D, Hull L, Moorthy K, et al. Self versus expert assessment of technical and non-technical skills in high-fidelity simulation. *Am J Surg.* 2011;202(4):500–506.
11. Flin R, Yule S, McKenzie L, Paterson-Brown S, Maran N. Attitudes to teamwork and safety in the operating theatre. *Surgeon.* 2006;4(3):145–151.
12. Makary MA, Sexton JB, Freischlag JA, et al. Operating room teamwork among physicians and nurses: teamwork in the eye of the beholder. *J Am Coll Surg.* 2006;202(5):746–752.
13. Yule S, Flin R, Paterson-Brown S, Maran N. Non-technical skills for surgeons in the operating room: a review of the literature. *Surgery.* 2006;139(2):140–149.
14. Yule S, Flin R, Maran N, Rowley D, Youngson G, Paterson-Brown S. Surgeons' non-technical skills in the operating room: reliability testing of the NOTSS behavior rating system. *World J Surg.* 2008;32(4):548–556.
15. Yule S, Rowley D, Flin R, Maran N, et al. Experience matters: comparing novice and expert ratings of non-technical skills using the NOTSS system. *ANZ J Surg.* 2009;79(3):154–160.
16. Sevdalis N, Davis R, Koutantji M, Undre S, Darzi A, Vincent CA. Reliability of a revised NOTECHS scale for use in surgical teams. *Am J Surg.* 2008;196(2):184–190.
17. Murray WB, Foster PA. Crisis resource management among strangers: principles of organizing a multidisciplinary group for crisis resource management. *J Clin Anesth.* 2000;12(8):633–638.
18. Paige JT. Surgical team training: promoting high reliability with non-technical skills. *Surg Clin North Am.* 2010;90(3):569–581.
19. Gaba DM, Howard SK, Fish KJ, Smith BE, Sowb YA. Simulation-based training in anesthesia crisis resource management (ACRM): A decade of experience. *Simulation and Gaming.* 2001;32:175–193.
20. Wilson KA, Burke CS, Priest HA, Salas E. Promoting healthcare safety through training high reliability teams. *Qual Saf Health Care.* 2005;14(4):303–339.

21. McGaghie WC, Issenberg SB, Petrusa ER, Scalese RJ. A critical review of simulation-based medical education research: 2003–2009. *Med Educ.* 2010;44(1):50–63.
22. Gettman MT, Pereira CW, Lipsky K, Wilson T, Arnold JJ, Leibovich BC, et al. Use of high-fidelity operating room simulation to assess and teach communication, teamwork and laparoscopic skills: initial experience. *J Urol.* 2009;181(3):1289–1296.
23. Powers KA, Rehrig ST, Irias N, et al. Simulated laparoscopic operating room crisis: an approach to enhance the surgical team performance. *Surg Endosc.* 2008;22(4):885–900.
24. Undre S, Koutantji M, Sevdalis N, et al. Multidisciplinary crisis simulations: the way forward for training surgical teams. *World J Surg.* 2007;31(9):1843–1853.
25. Paige JT, Kozmenko V, Yang T, et al. Attitudinal changes resulting from repetitive training of operating room personnel using of high-fidelity simulation at the point of care. *Am Surg.* 2009;75(7):584–590; discussion 90–91.
26. Fanning RM, Gaba DM. The role of debriefing in simulation-based learning. *Simul Healthc.* 2007;2(2):115–125.
27. Ahmed K, Amer T, Challacombe B, Jaye P, Dasgupta P, Khan MS. How to develop a simulation programme in urology. *BJU Int.* 2011;108(11):1698–1702.
28. Kirkpatrick DL. *Evaluating Training Programmes: The Four Levels.* San Francisco, CA: Berrett-Koehler; 1994.
29. Paige JT, Kozmenko V, Yang T, et al. High-fidelity, simulation-based, interdisciplinary operating room team training at the point of care. *Surgery.* 2009;145(2):138–146.
30. Gaba DM. Improving anesthesiologists' performance by simulating reality. *Anesthesiology.* 1992;76(4):491–494.
31. Haynes AB, Weiser TG, Berry WR, et al. A surgical safety checklist to reduce morbidity and mortality in a global population. *N Engl J Med.* 2009;360(5):491–499.
32. Wetzel CM, George A, Hanna GB, et al. Stress management training for surgeons: a randomized, controlled, intervention study. *Ann Surg.* 2011;253(3):488–494.
33. Riley R, ed. *Manual of Simulation in Healthcare.* New York: Oxford University Press; 2008.
34. UK. Parliament. House of Commons Health Committee (2009). *Patient Safety.* 6th report of the 2008–2009 session. http://www.publications.parliament.uk/pa/cm200809/cmselect/cmhealth/151/151i.pdf. Accessed 12 December 2013.

Chapter 6

LEARNING CURVES FOR SIMULATORS

Daniel A. Hashimoto and Rajesh Aggarwal

Five Key Messages

1. The learning curve plots improvement in surgical performance as a function of increasing experience.
2. Individuals progress along the learning curve at different rates.
3. Simulation training can decrease the length of the learning curve for trainees prior to entering the operating room.
4. Proficiency-based rather than time- or case-based simulation curricula are most effective in ensuring that individuals meet learning goals.
5. Effective simulation training is a cost-effective measure for teaching trainees surgical skills.

Defining the Learning Curve

The learning curve, described as the change in rate of learning in a specific task for the average individual, was first described in 1885 by German psychologist Hermann Ebbinghaus in his studies of human memory (1). Ebbinghaus's characterisation of the learning curve was based on his observation that the time required to perform verbal tasks increased as the task difficulty increased. The first mathematical model of the learning curve was developed to illustrate work productivity in aviation when Wright determined that as the production of aircraft increased, cost decreased (2). The learning curve model has since been broadened to describe the decrease in cost, be it financial, temporal, physical or mental, associated with the increased repetitions of a task.

Within surgical education, the concept of a learning curve has been described for both real and simulated operative procedures, showing improvement of technical skill as a function of procedural repetition (3–6). As in other fields, initial improvement can be quite rapid, but improvements slowly taper toward an asymptote often described as a 'plateau' in skill acquisition (7) (Figure 6.1). Interest in applying learning curves to surgical education is founded in efforts to maximise the efficiency of training while maintaining patient safety as the top priority. Efforts to define the metric by which the surgical learning curve should be measured have included plotting operative time and incidence of adverse outcomes as a function of operative experience (8).

Measuring the learning curve

There are multiple statistical tools available to demonstrate learning curves in operative procedures with some being more robust and appropriate than others. Different analyses can be employed depending on the preferences and requirements of the investigator, and those most relevant to surgical education are summarised briefly.

One of the simplest methods of demonstrating a learning curve involves arbitrarily dividing operative experience in a case series into groupings such as thirds or quartiles. The means of each group are then compared using a test of means (e.g., t-test, ANOVA) with learning considered to have occurred if differences are significant. This method of analysis is limited to demonstrating whether or not learning has occurred. Because performance means are analysed in arbitrary groups, one cannot identify specifically where on the curve learning plateaus or peak learning rates occur.

A more sophisticated method of looking at learning curves involves the analysis of repeated measures, either through ANOVA or its nonparametric equivalent, the Friedman test. These tests allow for the comparison of multiple means of performance across time to identify changes in the level of skill. Thus the analysis allows for identification of significant changes in performance from repetition to repetition, enabling investigators to identify learning plateaus on the learning curve.

Regression analysis encompasses a range of statistical methodologies (e.g., logistic, probit, least squares, etc.) that can be used to examine the relationship between measures of performance as a function of experience. It is useful not only for identifying learning plateaus, but also to estimate the rate of learning at different points along the learning curve. Regression analysis can be used to predict events by generating a best fit curve from available data and has been used to produce learning curves for surgery in both the simulated and operative settings (8, 9).

The cumulative sum chart (CUSUM) is a sequential analysis that can highlight small changes to the means of a process. CUSUM involves summing the differences between measured values and a benchmark value to determine the extent of deviation away from the benchmark. A threshold for change in both positive and negative value away from the benchmark is calculated. The CUSUM method can reliably provide information on when performance begins to either decline or improve outside of statistical expectations (10).

Investigators select different methods to determine the learning curve based on experience and need (9). Comparisons of arbitrary groups can demonstrate absolute changes in performance but is otherwise limited in its utility. Repeated measures and regression analyses allow for the identification of specific points of learning plateau along the curve while CUSUM is best utilised for monitoring performance of a trainee's educational progression and to identify when remediation may be necessary (6).

The learning curve in the operating room

The advent of laparoscopy and other minimally invasive techniques has been driving an interest in investigating the relationship between case volume and outcome. In 1995, the Southern Surgeons Club conducted a large prospective study of over 8,839 cases by 55 surgeons to investigate the learning curve in laparoscopic cholecystectomy (LC), with a patient follow-up time of six months. Regression analysis in the study assessed the chance of bile duct injury as a function of different measured variables and showed that only the surgeon's experience in LC was significantly associated with adverse outcome ($p = 0.001$).

The learning curve shows that for a surgeon with no experience in LC, a 1.7% chance of bile duct injury can be expected, with the risk of bile duct injury decreasing to 0.48% after 10 cases, 0.31% after 20 cases and 0.17% after 50 cases. This study not only demonstrates that the chance of bile duct injury can be reduced by 90% through increased surgical experience but also illustrates the learning curve effect of increased operative experience leading to decreased incidence of adverse outcomes (8).

Similar learning curve studies have been conducted in other surgical subspecialties. CUSUM analysis of laparoscopic colectomy demonstrated an increased conversion to open rates until the 55th case for right-sided colectomy and the 62nd case for left-sided colectomy. On average there is a 5.1-fold increased risk of conversion to open in laparoscopic colectomy in the first 25 cases and a 3.8-fold increased risk in the 25th to 50th cases compared to conversion rate after 175 cases (11). Learning curves also apply to robotic procedures such as robotic prostatectomy. One literature review found that proficiency is suggested to occur between 20 and 25 cases, however, for outcomes similar to radical retropubic prostatectomy, over 150 cases of experience in robotic prostatectomy may be needed (12).

While trainees must obtain experience to become more skilled at performing procedures, the necessity of education must be considered in the context of patient safety. Due to increased awareness of the learning curve, surgical education has shifted away from the classic 'see one and do one and teach one' apprenticeship model to a more safety-driven model that incorporates the use of surgical simulators into training with the aim of reducing the learning curve for surgeons in a standardised controlled setting outside of the operating room.

Reducing the learning curve

Technological advances have allowed for the development of simulators beyond simple cadaveric animal tissue or expensive anaesthetised live animals. Inanimate trainers are available in many forms and offer varying degrees of fidelity. Trainers such as the Fundamentals of Laparoscopic Surgery (FLS) box offer trainees the ability to perform basic laparoscopic tasks on simple objects such as ropes and pegs (13). Others utilise more complex and arguably more realistic representations of anatomy to simulate portions of entire procedures such as laparoscopic appendectomy and cholecystectomy.

Virtual reality (VR) simulators allow surgeons to practise procedures in a computer-generated environment and provide the advantage of having built-in, automated measures of assessment such as motion and dexterity parameters on standardised educational modules. While the initial cost of investment in VR simulators can be high, subsequent maintenance is relatively inexpensive. Furthermore, trainees can receive instruction from modules built into the simulators, allowing them to practise skills independent of a proctor or instructor if necessary (14).

The importance of incorporating simulators into surgical training has been recognised by governing bodies such as the Residency Review Committee of the Accreditation Council for Graduate Medical Education (ACGME) in the United States, which mandated in 2008 that all American surgical residency programmes have access to a simulation laboratory with the aim that incorporating simulation into training would reduce the length of the learning curve before trainees operate on live patients (15).

Simulation-based learning curves and simulator curricula

Multiple studies have provided evidence for the transfer of skills acquired in the simulation centre to actual procedures in the operating room, suggesting that simulation training may contribute to the acquisition of experience necessary to advance along the learning curve (16, 17). Therefore, it is important to understand that optimal performance on a simulator is also subject to a learning curve.

Feldman et al. described the learning curve for the peg transfer task in the FLS box trainer, part of a minimally invasive curriculum mandatory for surgical trainees in the United States (6). Through nonlinear regression, inverse learning curves were fit to the performance of the task for each of the 16 medical students over 40 repetitions. The 'learning plateau' was defined as the asymptote of the learning curve and represented a 'theoretical best score [that could be achieved] with infinite practice'. Over the course of 40 repetitions, the average score per trial improved as a function of practice with baseline scores (out of 100) of 48 ± 24 improving to 94 ± 8 by the 40th repetition. The mean learning plateau was estimated at 89.6 ± 9.6, and the study found that the learning rates were highly variable between subjects, consistent with observations that learning curves vary for different individuals.

The MIST-VR simulator (Mentice Inc., Gothenburg, Sweden) is one of the first and the most well validated virtual reality laparoscopic simulators (7, 18, 19). It provides 12 tasks representative of various laparoscopic skills at three difficulty levels. Brunner et al. conducted a study to investigate the learning curves for each task on the MIST-VR, plotting mean scores for each task as a function of the number of repetitions (7). An initial plateau in performance was demonstrated to have developed by the eighth repetition for all tasks; but, continued repetition of tasks led to an ultimate plateau in performance between the 21th and 30th repetition (Table 6.1).

Such studies demonstrate the learning curve in surgical simulation, and simulation has been shown to shorten the length of the learning curve for real procedures in the operating room when compared to no simulation training (20). The study by Feldman et al. demonstrates the concern that merely performing a predetermined number of cases may not be sufficient to obtain competency given the variability in individual learning curves (6). For effective simulation-based education, proficiency-based curricula should be utilised to ensure individual competency.

Proficiency-based curricula

While many commercially available VR simulators come with pre-programmed curricula and suggested performance metrics, suggestions are rarely based on studies validating their use for effective surgical training. The following curricula incorporate construct valid tasks, i.e., tasks that can distinguish the performance of novices from experienced surgeons to advance novice surgeons along the learning curve to a benchmark level of proficiency.

MIST-VR curriculum

The structured curriculum of skills acquisition on the MIST-VR was developed by investigating the learning curves of 20 medical students on 12 tasks. Trainees progress through all 12 tasks first at easy and then medium difficulty, where plateaus in the learning curve typically occurred between sessions two and six. The skills acquired at easy and medium difficulty over repeated practice should then translate to specific performance targets at the hard difficulty level where assessment of skill can occur against an expert-derived performance standard (21). The performance-based criteria for skill proficiency takes into account the fact that different learners will progress at different rates along the learning curve; thus, the amount of time or number of repetitions required to complete the programme is irrelevant as some learners will progress through the learning curve more quickly than others and hit performance targets sooner.

LapSim curriculum

Using the model of the MIST-VR curriculum, a similar validated curriculum for the LapSim VR simulator (Surgical Science, Gothenburg, Sweden), which has seven basic tasks at three difficulty levels, has been developed. Construct validity is demonstrated for all seven tasks using time taken and path length as metrics, and learning curves plateaued at a median of seven repetitions for all tasks. Benchmark parameters for novices to attain proficiency were set at the median score for the experienced surgeons after two sessions (22).

LAP Mentor curriculum

Aggarwal et al. developed an evidence-based curriculum for training to proficiency in laparoscopic cholecystectomy using the LAP Mentor VR simulator (Simbionix Corporation, Cleveland, Ohio, USA) (23). Construct valid metrics all showed significant learning curves, with plateaus in performance at the seventh repetition, as measured by time taken, total number of movements, total cautery time and total cautery time without tissue contact for dissection of Calot's triangle. This validated curriculum also uses validated performance targets for proficiency rather than the time spent practicing tasks.

As evidenced by the three examples of curricular validation, development of a competency-based curriculum requires the identification of construct valid tasks and performance-based rather than time- or repetition-based criteria for completion. Performance-based curricula for the attainment of proficiency account for different rates of learning in individuals and ensure that trainees are truly acquiring an acceptable level of skill prior to performing procedures on real patients.

Curricula can be built upon a framework for the systematic training and assessment of technical skills (STATS) (14). STATS addresses technical skills training from early acquisition to finally granting privileges for practice by providing a roadmap to guide the development of a curriculum to address education along the learning curve. Early education focuses on knowledge-based learning and advances to providing an understanding of the deconstructed portions of a procedure that can be practiced on a validated model. These skills can then be assessed as they translate to the real operating room, culminating in a final assessment to advance the trainee to independent practice.

Transfer effectiveness ratio

The goal of simulation is to shorten the learning curve for real procedures so that trainees can safely and effectively transition their education from the simulation centre to the operating room. The effectiveness of a simulator can thus be assessed using the transfer effectiveness ratio (TER), first utilised by the aviation industry to assess the efficacy of virtual flight simulators in decreasing the learning curve of piloting real aircraft (24, 25).

TER is calculated as

- TER = $(X_1 - X_2)/T$

where:

- X_1 = median time required by non-simulator-trained group to reach performance criteria;
- X_2 = median time required to achieve performance criterion in simulator-trained group;
- T = total training time of the simulator-trained group (20).

TER is a useful measure to determine the amount of training time that can be saved by utilizing simulation within a curriculum. For example, a TER of two would suggest that every minute spent training on a simulator is equivalent to two minutes training on the comparative model. In the context of surgical education, TER has been utilised to assess the efficacy of simulators such as the LapSim VR laparoscopic simulator where TER for proficiency training was found to be 2.28 (20). TER calculation can be affected by the performance criteria set for users. For example, Kolozsvari et al. found the TER of the FLS peg transfer task to be 0.16 when targeting a 'mastery' level of performance in preparation for learning intracorporeal suturing (26).

Conclusions

The adoption of novel surgical technologies and techniques requires surgeons to develop an increasingly diverse set of technical skills in a time- and cost-efficient manner. Simulation allows trainees to address difficulties in spatial awareness and psychomotor dexterity prior to advancing to more complex skills; thus, initial basic training in the skills laboratory can shorten the learning curve for more advanced procedures while decreasing the cost of training (27, 28). Given studies investigating the TER of laparoscopic simulators, investing trainee time in simulation learning may improve the efficiency of knowledge transfer in laparoscopy if structured, proficiency-based curricula are properly utilised. As technology continues to be integrated into modern surgical curricula, an awareness of the learning curve for skills acquisition can guide efficient, effective surgical training.

Figures and Tables

Figure 6.1. The traditional learning curve demonstrating the decrease in incidence of adverse events as experience increases

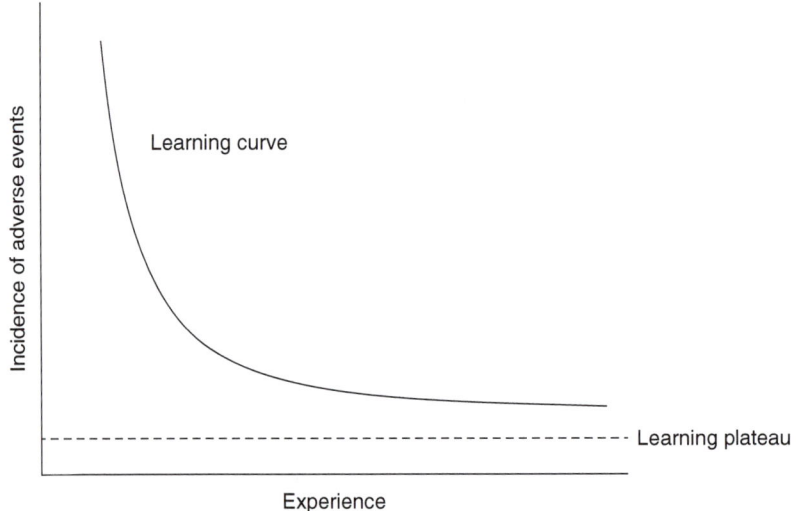

Table 6.1. Comparison of mean learning plateaus for novices in various virtual reality simulators

Simulator	Mean learning plateau reached
MIST-VR	8th repetition, 21st–30th repetition
LapSim	7th repetition
LAP Mentor	7th repetition

References

1. Ebbinghaus H. *Memory: A Contribution to Experimental Psychology*. New York: Teachers College, Columbia University; 1913. Repr. Bristol: Thoemmes Press; 1999.
2. Wright T. Factors affecting the cost of airplanes. *Journal of Aeronautical Sciences*. 1936;3(4)122–128.
3. Ahlberg G, et al. Is the learning curve for laparoscopic fundoplication determined by the teacher or the pupil? *Am J Surg*. 2005;189(2):184–189.
4. Senagore AJ, Luchtefeld MA, Mackeigan JM. What is the learning curve for laparoscopic colectomy? *Am J Surg*. 1995;61(8):681–685.
5. Club SS. A prospective analysis of 1,518 laparoscopic cholecystectomies. The Southern Surgeons Club. *N Engl J Med*. 1991;324(16):1073–1078.
6. Feldman LS, et al. A method to characterize the learning curve for performance of a fundamental laparoscopic simulator task: defining 'learning plateau' and 'learning rate'. *Surgery*. 2009;146(2):381–386.
7. Brunner WC, et al. Laparoscopic virtual reality training: are 30 repetitions enough? *J Surg Res*. 2004;122(2):150–156.
8. Moore MJ, Bennett CL. The learning curve for laparoscopic cholecystectomy. The Southern Surgeons Club. *Am J Surg*. 1995;170(1):55–59.
9. Ramsay CR, et al. Statistical assessment of the learning curves of health technologies. *Health Technol Assess*. 2001;5(12):1–79.
10. NIST/SEMATECH. *e-Handbook of Statistical Methods*. http://www.itl.nist.gov/div898/handbook/. Accessed 12 December 2013.
11. Tekkis PP, et al. Evaluation of the learning curve in laparoscopic colorectal surgery: comparison of right-sided and left-sided resections. *Ann Surg*. 2005;242(1):83–91.
12. Freire MP, et al. Overcoming the learning curve for robotic-assisted laparoscopic radical prostatectomy. *Urol Clin North Am*. 2010;37(1):37–47, table of contents.
13. Peters JH, et al. Development and validation of a comprehensive program of education and assessment of the basic fundamentals of laparoscopic surgery. *Surgery*. 2004;135(1):21–27.

14. Aggarwal R, Grantcharov TP, and Darzi A. Framework for systematic training and assessment of technical skills. *J Am Coll Surg*. 2007;204(4): 697–705.
15. ACGME. ACGME Program Requirements of Graduate Medical Education in Surgery. R. R. Committee, ed. Chicago, IL: Accreditation Council for Graduate Medical Education; 2008.
16. Seymour NE, et al. Virtual reality training improves operating room performance: results of a randomized, double-blinded study. *Ann Surg*. 2002;236(4):458–463, discussion 463–464.
17. Hamilton EC, et al. Improving operative performance using a laparoscopic hernia simulator. *Am J Surg*. 2001;182(6):725–728.
18. Aggarwal R, et al. A competency-based virtual reality training curriculum for the acquisition of laparoscopic psychomotor skill. *Am J Surg*. 2006;191(1):128–133.
19. Chaudhry A, et al. Learning rate for laparoscopic surgical skills on MIST-VR™, a virtual reality simulator: quality of human–computer interface. *Ann R Coll Surg Engl*. 1999;81(4):281–286.
20. Aggarwal R, et al. Proving the effectiveness of virtual reality simulation for training in laparoscopic surgery. *Ann Surg*. 2007;246(5):771–779.
21. Gallagher AG, et al. Psychomotor skills assessment in practicing surgeons experienced in performing advanced laparoscopic procedures. *J Am Coll Surg*. 2003;197(3):479–488.
22. Aggarwal R, et al. An evidence-based virtual reality training program for novice laparoscopic surgeons. *Ann Surg*. 2006;244(2):310–314.
23. Aggarwal R, et al. Development of a virtual reality training curriculum for laparoscopic cholecystectomy. *Br J Surg*. 2009;96(9):1086–1093.
24. Roscoe SN. A little more on incremental transfer effectiveness. *Human Factors*. 1972;14(4):363–367.
25. Roscoe SN. Incremental Transfer Effectiveness. *Human Factors*. 1971;13(6):561–567.
26. Kolozsvari NO, et al. Mastery versus the standard proficiency target for basic laparoscopic skill training: effect on skill transfer and retention. *Surg Endosc*. 2011;25(7):2063–2070.
27. Stefanidis D, et al. Initial laparoscopic basic skills training shortens the learning curve of laparoscopic suturing and is cost-effective. *J Am Coll Surg*. 2010;210(4):436–440.
28. Scott DJ, et al. Laparoscopic training on bench models: better and more cost effective than operating room experience? *J Am Coll Surg*. 2000;191(3):272–283.

Chapter 7

DEVELOPING A SIMULATION PROGRAMME

Kamran Ahmed, Fahd Khan, Nuzhath Khan, Mohammed Shamim Khan and Prokar Dasgupta

Introduction

Urology training has traditionally adopted an apprenticeship model whereby trainees are taught and overseen by senior surgeons in clinical settings and operating theatres. This method has thus far produced safe and competent surgeons. Although the operating theatre is regarded as the best learning resource, it is difficult to balance the benefit of learning from exposure to real patients with the potential harm to these patients if operated on by trainee surgeons. Also, the operating theatre is a stressful environment with time constraints and numerous distractions, making it a less than ideal stage for learning. To add to these challenges, trainees and trained surgeons alike must adapt to emerging innovations in urology such as laparoscopic and robotic technologies, which have steep learning curves. Furthermore, the reduction in trainee working hours and a shorter training period means that the largely opportunity-based apprenticeship model of training alone is no longer sufficient. Thus, the traditional urology training programme faces a number of challenges: providing ample learning opportunities with novel technologies in authentic environments without compromising patient safety, and within a shorter training period.

The use of simulators and inanimate trainers addresses many of these challenges. Simulators are products that mimic realistic tasks and situations in a controlled setting. Many types of simulations exist, from synthetic, animal and cadaveric organ models to mechanical and virtual reality simulators (a computer-generated representation of realistic environments that allow user interaction). Simulators provide the opportunity to practise the necessary skills in a controlled environment without compromising patient safety. The stresses and time constraints of the operating theatre are removed, creating a safe and predictable environment in which to develop skills which have been shown to be transferable to the operating theatre (1). Virtual programmes provide ample opportunity to become familiar with novel technologies such as laparoscopic and robotic procedures (2). Practice and repetition in a controlled environment reduces the learning curve for skills acquisition (3).

There are many considerations that must be taken into account when developing a simulation programme. Some of these will be discussed below and include which factors to consider in the choice of simulators to be used in the programme, issues regarding space and finance, the importance of leadership, a successful integration into curricula and, finally, some challenges including the lack of research into the validity of simulators.

Deciding Which Simulators to Use

Deciding which simulators to use is an important step in developing a simulation programme. It is helpful to decide which procedures would benefit most from simulated training. Procedures that are complex, high risk to patients and have steep learning curves are good candidates for simulation. For example, the use of robotic and laparoscopic technology is becoming increasingly popular within urology. These complex procedures tend to have steeper learning curves and would therefore benefit from practice and repetition with a simulator. High-fidelity laparoscopic virtual simulators such as the Minimally Invasive Surgical Trainer (MIST) and LAP Mentor have been developed for this purpose. From an industry perspective, other factors such as the frequency with which the procedure is performed and the number of trainees that are likely to use the simulator may gain priority (4). Common procedures that are frequently performed such as transurethral resection of the prostate (TURP), a technique most urologists are required to master, have been chosen for simulation.

Having decided on the procedures that may benefit most from simulated training, it may be helpful to understand the learning steps that lead to mastering a procedure. A group of basic skills are first acquired that, when chained together, make up a particular task; and when a string of tasks are combined, they form the basis of a procedure. For example, basic tasks such as instrument handling and knot tying comprise tasks such as suturing and tissue dissection which form the basis of procedures such as appendicectomy (Figure 7.1) (5). This helps group different simulators into categories; for example, those that help acquire basic skills as opposed to intermediate tasks and partial or complete procedures. A simulation programme must at least have the simulators that aid the learning of basic skills and then tasks and ultimately procedures.

Basic skills and tasks such as clipping/cutting, dissection, object manipulation and suturing can be practised on box/video trainers and synthetic and animal tissue models, but whole procedures such as laparoscopic procedures can be practised on virtual reality simulators. However, simulators that train basic skills such as box trainers have low fidelity compared to virtual reality simulators. Thus it is important to consider the level of 'realism' of the simulator, i.e., the extent to which it replicates the real task or situation. Levels of realism including visual, physical, physiological and tactile realism have been described (Table 7.1) (4). The simulator must visually mimic a realistic scenario, be physically and dynamically interactive with the user, replicate the physiological properties of tissues and organs and provide tactile feedback to manipulation. Simulators with high levels of realism are described as having high fidelity.

The advantage of such high-fidelity simulators is that they are able to move beyond basic skills training to more complex and complete procedures. Examples include animal and cadaveric models and some high-fidelity virtual reality simulators. However, animal models are costly, not readily available and raise ethical concerns. In contrast, low-fidelity simulators such as mechanical box trainers and some virtual reality simulators are low cost and have been shown to be as beneficial as high-fidelity simulators in terms of skills acquisition and transfer (6, 7). Studies have shown that there is no difference in skills acquisition when high-fidelity virtual reality trainers are substituted for box trainers and that both provide equal improvement in basic surgical skills (8, 9). Thus, the goal is to find the level of realism and fidelity that fits the task and allows the maximum level of skills transfer, and the point at which additional increase in transfer is not worth the added costs.

Funding and Financial Issues

One of the major obstacles in developing a simulation programme is the large capital required in the initial start-up and running of the programme. These initial costs include premises, personnel and training materials. Adequate physical space is required to successfully set up a skills lab, which may include a task training room, simulation room, control and observer centre and conference room (5). A full-time technical employee may need to be hired for set-up and scheduling, equipment upkeep, tracking attendance and so on. Cost of purchase of simulators and supporting training materials is of course mandatory. Funding can be obtained from a variety of sources including public (such as the hospital or surgical department budget) and private or philanthropic sources (such as industry or alumni) (5, 10).

In the face of the current financial climate, it is essential to consider ways to minimise the costs of running a simulation programme. One idea is to liaise with other surgical departments to share resources. Communication between different departments may reveal shared interests that may be used to plan collaboratively the use of resources. Research has shown that skills laboratories that share resources are able to attain more equipment including video trainers and virtual reality trainers, perhaps through saving on other costs such as space (10). It has also been suggested that the dynamic costs of running a simulation programme, such as the ongoing purchase of supporting materials (i.e., suturing material and laparoscopic instruments), can be reduced by liaising with operating theatres across departments to donate discontinued and expired products (11). Communication between simulation programmes need not be restricted to departments within an institution but expanded across various institutions. The ideal simulation programme would have a mix of high- and low-fidelity simulators to match various learning requirements. However, in reality, very few centres can afford the high-fidelity virtual reality simulators. One suggestion has been to develop a hub-and-spoke service model where a larger, centralised simulation centre with better investments and a larger repertoire of simulators can liaise with peripheral centres in order to share resources (12).

Another way in which cost can be minimised is by the appropriate planning and scheduling of the simulation programme to maximise usage. It has been suggested that use of the simulation programme should be mandatory (11). Many institutions have taken this approach, which has led to increased utilisation and funding from several resources (10). It is difficult to justify the high cost of running a simulation centre without adequate usage. As well as providing justification for spending, mandatory usage allows effective planning and scheduling as participation numbers can be predicted. Overall, this ensures easier integration into the curriculum.

Leadership and Management

In order to thrive, a simulation programme requires strong leadership. Faculty member participation should be strongly encouraged by department and programme leaders (5). Ideally, leaders of the programme should be members who are urologists (12). This helps in promoting the agenda of simulation and setting the tone for trainee participations. Often these individuals have high credibility and connections and are in a good position to negotiate funding from public and private sources (12). Simulation programmes require at least one dedicated full-time faculty member who is willing to devote time to the managing of the centre as well as acting as a skills coach. It has been suggested that faculty members with experience in clinical teaching maximise the benefit of training programmes (11). However, time constraints and lack of financial reward and recognition for simulation teaching and educational research may deter many faculty members from full commitment. In order to engage faculty, institutions must recognise and reward teaching and educational research. This has been done in a number of institutions through teaching incentive schemes and incorporating teaching into promotion and tenure (11).

Integration into Curricula

In order to maximise the benefits of a simulation programme, it should not be portrayed as a standalone resource but as part of a well-structured curriculum. However, this is not an easy task and many organisations have struggled with it (13). One issue is that curriculum content and design varies widely between institutions. Much of the educational literature supports the need to create a national standardised curriculum with proficiency-based strategies (14, 15). It has been suggested that surgeons acquire technical skills by a series of steps. The trainee first cognitively orientates themselves to the mechanics of the task by observing a demonstration. This is followed by practice and repetition of the task until it can be carried out with fluidity and, finally, proficiency is achieved when the task can be demonstrated autonomously, without thinking, and attention can be focused beyond the mechanics of the task (14). A validated simulation programme can be used to support and implement such a proficiency-based curriculum as it has inbuilt objective measures of assessment from which proficiency levels can be derived.

This has been shown in the work of Aggarwal et al., who have designed a proficiency-based curriculum for basic laparoscopic skills acquisition (15). Performance criteria were preset by pooling the scores of expert surgeons on the simulator. Thus benchmark proficiency criteria were defined for endpoints for each task such as time taken, number of errors and path lengths. This created the basis of a proficiency-based curriculum with clearly defined endpoints. Progression along the curriculum could be charted by passing set performance criteria so proficiency can be defined. The curricula could commence by defining baseline knowledge and teaching basic skills on low-fidelity bench simulators before progressing to more complex skills on virtual reality simulators. Time limits could be given for achieving proficiency in certain tasks. Objective assessments such as end-of-module examinations should be carried out to assure competency targets are being met. Friedell has described a proficiency-based curriculum whereby trainees undergo baseline assessment, self practice with deadlines to ensure expert derived proficiency levels are met within a certain time frame and final assessments to ensure suitable skills acquisition (5).

It can be argued that proficiency at the level of a simulator does not necessarily translate to proficiency in the operating theatre. However, research indicates that performance-based simulated curricula have led to effective skills acquisition and improved operating theatre performance. For example, proficiency-based simulator training in laparoscopic suturing and knot tying improved performance in the operating room (16, 17). Furthermore, a proficiency-based simulator curriculum ensures uniform skills acquisition by ensuring all trainees reach a set level of competency. Thus a well-structured performance-based curriculum with well-defined endpoints and benchmark criteria is crucial to the development of a simulation programme.

Challenges

There are a few challenges involved in the successful development of a simulation programme, some of which have already been discussed. There are large initial costs in setting up a programme, including the establishment of premises, personnel and equipment. There are issues with recruiting full-time, dedicated faculty members who will act as leaders and skills coaches and promote the use of the programme. However, one major challenge is the lack of evidence and research into the effectiveness of simulators and their validity (especially predictive validity).

Before a simulator can be introduced into training and incorporated into a simulation programme, it must be tested for reliability and validity. A reliable simulator performs consistently in the same manner with both single and variable observers on different occasions. In broad terms, validity measures whether the simulator performs the functions that it was intended to perform. Various benchmarks have been developed to assess validity such as face, content, construct, concurrent and predictive validity (Table 7.2) (18). Face validity subjectively measures performance at face value; content validity reviews each component of the programme to test whether it is appropriate and useful; construct validity tests whether the programme can distinguish between expert and novice performance; concurrent validity measures whether performance from the programme correlates well with performance from the existing training method; and predictive validity measures the degree to which performance at the simulator predicts future performance in the real environment (18–20).

For example, studies have measured the face, content and construct validity of the virtual reality simulator, da Vinci Si Surgeon Console and Mimic.

Three groups of participants (novice, intermediate and expert) rated the level of realism (face validity) and training usefulness (content validity) of the simulator via questionnaire. Performance measures of the three groups on the simulator were compared, measuring construct validity (21). In a later study, the same simulator was tested for concurrent and predictive validity by showing a high correlation of performance with robotic surgical performance (concurrent validity) and future performance (predictive validity) on animal tissue models (22).

Although the aforementioned benchmark criteria for establishing validity all have merit, predictive validity is the one most likely to be clinically relevant. Face and content validity are largely subjective and rely on trainee self reports and expert opinion. In an ideal simulator with good predictive validity, scores measured on the simulator would predict performance in the operating theatre. For example, studies have shown that performance scores from some simulators correlate well with assessment of the performance in the operating theatre after a period of time (23, 24). Although it is regarded as the ideal benchmark, predictive validity is not frequently measured. The relative ease with which face and content validity can be measured in comparison to predictive validity, which requires a long-term follow up, may explain this. A recent systematic review found that out of 83 studies about the validation of simulators, only 5% measured predictive validity (the majority measured construct (60%) and concurrent (24%) validity, and less than half reported reliability) (25).

However, without strong evidence of validity, in particular predictive validity, it is difficult to justify the use of simulators for training, especially with the high costs involved. Therefore, we need further research into and evidence of the validity of simulators, especially due to the high rate at which new programmes are being introduced into the market.

Conclusion

Simulation is beginning to play a more important role in surgical education. This is largely due to reduced working hours and a shorter training period, resulting in a lack of opportunities to practise vital skills safely in a clinical setting, in particular with complex emerging technologies. However, there are many considerations in designing a simulation programme including choosing the right simulator, cost, management and integration into curricula. Simulators should be suited to the level of training and chosen appropriately so that they build up from basic skills to complex procedures. Decisions regarding the cost versus fidelity of the simulator must be made. The cost of running a training programme can be reduced by sharing resources with other departments and creating larger, centralised centres for the use of high-fidelity simulators. Careful scheduling and mandatory involvement maximises use of the programme and justifies cost. Faculty members should be rewarded for involvement with teaching and research into simulation and full-time involvement should be encouraged. Simulators should be fully integrated into a proficiency-based curriculum with set performance criteria and objective assessment. Research into the validation of simulators for use in programmes is encouraged.

Figures and Tables

Figure 7.1. Surgical simulators can be used to build up from basic skills to tasks and finally procedures (5)

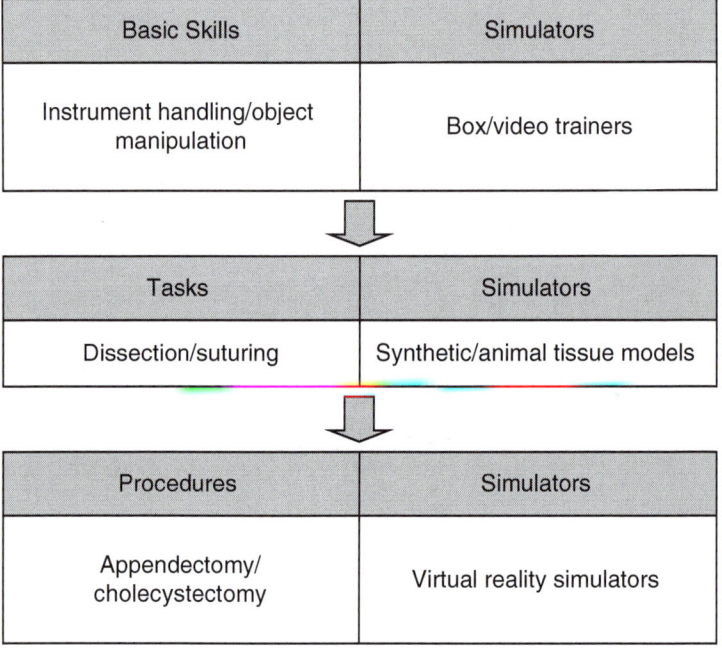

DEVELOPING A SIMULATION PROGRAMME

Table 7.1. Levels of 'realism' or fidelity of simulators (4)

Visual realism	The simulator must look realistic or visually represent a real environment.
Physical realism	The simulator must allow direct physical interaction with the user and respond realistically to physical forces and manipulation.
Physiological realism	The simulator must realistically replicate the physiological properties of tissues such as bleeding or bruising in response to manipulation.
Tactile realism	The simulator must provide tactile feedback to the user in response to manipulation.

Table 7.2. Benchmarks for assessment of validity of simulators (18)

Face validity	A very subjective type of validity that measures whether the simulator seems to measure what it is supposed to. This can be derived from expert and novice user review and opinion.
Content validity	Again, slightly subjective; expert and novice users may provide their opinion of the usefulness and relevance of the simulator based on its content.
Construct validity	This measures the ability of the simulator to differentiate between expert and novice performance (i.e., whether it can test and identify the skills it was designed to measure).
Concurrent validity	This measures whether performance from the simulator is concurrent with performance from another previously validated training method.
Predictive validity	This measures whether performance at the simulator is predictive of performance in the non-simulated environment (e.g., the operating theatre) at a later point in time.

References

1. Sturm LP, Windsor JA, Cosman PH, et al. A systematic review of skills transfer after surgical simulation training. *Ann Surg.* 2008;248(2):166–179.
2. Gurusamy KS, Aggarwal R, Palanivelu L, Davidson BR. Virtual reality training for surgical trainees in laparoscopic surgery. *Cochrane Database Syst Rev.* 2009;(1)CD006575.
3. Aggarwal R, Ward J, Balasundaram I, et al. Proving the effectiveness of virtual reality simulation for training in laparoscopic surgery. *Ann Surg.* 2007;246(5):771–779.
4. Stacey RL. Marketing medical simulation: what industry needs from the clinical community. *Min Invas Ther & Allied Technol.* 2000;9(5):357–360.
5. Friedell ML. Starting a simulation and skills laboratory: what do I need and what do I want? *J Surg Educ.* 2010;67(2):112–121.
6. Shah J, Mackay S, Vale J, Darzi A. Simulation in urology: a role for virtual reality? *BJU Int.* 2001;88(7):661–665.
7. Wignall GR, Denstedt JD, Preminger GM, et al. Surgical simulation: a urological perspective. *J Urol.* 2008 May;179(5):1690–1699.
8. Madan AK, Frantzides CT. Substituting virtual reality trainers for inanimate box trainers does not decrease laparoscopic skills acquisition. *JSLS.* 2007;11(1):87–89.
9. Debes AJ, Aggarwal R, Balasundaram I, Jacobsen MB. A tale of two trainers: virtual reality versus a video trainer for acquisition of basic laparoscopic skills. *Am J Surg.* 2010;199(6):840–845.
10. Gould JC. Building a laparoscopic surgical skills training laboratory: resources and support. *JSLS.* 2006;10(3):293–296.
11. Bath J, Lawrence PF. Twelve tips for developing and implementing an effective surgical simulation programme. *Med Teach.* 2012;34(3):192–197.
12. Ahmed K, Amer T, Challacombe B, et al. How to develop a simulation programme in urology. *BJU Int.* 2011;108(11):1698–1702.
13. Meier AH. Running a surgical education center: from small to large. *Surg Clin North Am.* 2010;90(3):491–504.
14. McClusky DA, 3rd, Smith CD. Design and development of a surgical skills simulation curriculum. *World J Surg.* 2008;32(2):171–181.
15. Aggarwal R, Grantcharov TP, Eriksen JR, et al. An evidence-based virtual reality training program for novice laparoscopic surgeons. *Ann Surg.* 2006;244(2):310–314.
16. Stefanidis D, Acker C, Heniford BT. Proficiency-based laparoscopic simulator training leads to improved operating room skill that is resistant to decay. *Surg Innov.* 2008;15(1):69–73.

17. Korndorffer JR, Jr, Dunne JB, Sierra R, et al. Simulator training for laparoscopic suturing using performance goals translates to the operating room. *J Am Coll Surg*. 2005;201(1):23–29.
18. Gallagher AG, Ritter EM, Satava RM. Fundamental principles of validation, and reliability: rigorous science for the assessment of surgical education and training. *Surg Endosc*. 2003;17(10):1525–1529.
19. Schout BM, Hendrikx AJ, Scheele F, Bemelmans BL, Scherpbier AJ. Validation and implementation of surgical simulators: a critical review of present, past, and future. *Surg Endosc*. 2010;24(3):536–546.
20. McDougall EM. Validation of surgical simulators. *J Endourol*. 2007;21(3):244–247.
21. Hung AJ, Zehnder P, Patil MB, et al. Face, content and construct validity of a novel robotic surgery simulator. *J Urol*. 2011;186(3):1019–1024.
22. Hung AJ, Patil MB, Zehnder P, et al. Concurrent and predictive validation of a novel robotic surgery simulator: a prospective, randomized study. *J Urol*. 2012;187(2):630–637.
23. Fried GM, Feldman LS, Vassiliou MC, et al. Proving the value of simulation in laparoscopic surgery. *Ann Surg*. 2004;240(3):518–525; discussion 25–28.
24. Banks EH, Chudnoff S, Karmin I, Wang C, Pardanani S. Does a surgical simulator improve resident operative performance of laparoscopic tubal ligation? *Am J Obstet Gynecol*. 2007;197(5):541 e1–5.
25. Van Nortwick SS, Lendvay TS, Jensen AR, et al. Methodologies for establishing validity in surgical simulation studies. *Surgery*. 2010;147(5):622–630.

Chapter 8

PATIENT SAFETY AND SIMULATION

Ravindra Mehta, John Fitzpatrick and Ghulam Nabi

Introduction

Patient safety remains a major focus of modern healthcare. The US Institute of Medicine (IOM) report, *To Err is Human: Building a Safer Health System*, suggested that deaths due to medical errors exceed the total number of fatalities reported from motor vehicle accidents, breast cancer or AIDS, respectively (1). Some of the issues identified in this report could be addressed by adequately training the workforce in question. Training has traditionally always been acquired whilst treating live patients via the implementation of an 'on-the-job apprenticeship' model. This is unsatisfactory and has become virtually obsolete in the modern educational curriculum. Emphasis should therefore be laid upon initially training novices prior to their interaction with live patients in a patient-free environment using simulation, which risks no harm to patients.

Education has traditionally focused on imparting the knowledge necessary to practise medicine. However, modern training systems focus on the parameters of acceptable clinical practice within the framework of patient safety. Healthcare delivery is fast changing, especially with the introduction of new techniques in surgical practice. This highlights the importance of both a lifelong learning process and the introduction of simulation technology. Simulation is "a technique to replace or amplify real patient experiences with guided [experience that artificially] replicates substantial aspects of the real world in a fully interactive manner" (2). Simulation is designed to address the fast-changing needs of healthcare by providing a mosaic of technical and non-technical skills in a crawl–walk–run approach.

Simulation training in surgery is becoming embedded in the modern curriculum to further improve patient safety. This is driven by many factors including the desire of patients to avoid trainees 'practising' on them during their learning phase. There is good evidence that simulation training improves operational performance in the clinical setting, and data is still emerging to suggest that simulation actually improves patient outcome. The scope and practice of simulation in surgical education is growing, and this chapter aims to review the current literature to study simulation use in surgery and, in particular, its role in enhancing patient safety. Simulation technology could be used to build a 'safe, patient-centred culture' through changes at different levels in the delivery of care, specifically designed to change the human factors that influence people and their behaviour.

Pathogenesis of Unsafe Clinical Practice

Healthcare professionals, like any other human beings, are fallible and make mistakes, but the impact of most of these is not catastrophic. An increased awareness of such incidents often reduces the risk of such events.

An error in medical practice, as in any other organisational set up, is a manifestation of a breach in the multiple layers of defences known in healthcare as the 'Swiss cheese model' of incidents (Figure 8.1). Potential 'holes' exist in each of the defence levels, usually caused by poor management, less than acceptable decision making, inadequate resources, lack of training, stress, etc. These holes, also referred to as 'latent conditions', align together at successive levels of defences and create opportunities for unsafe practice or 'medical errors' to arise. It is evident that for any such error to happen, it is unlikely that any single action or failure would be responsible.

So, what leads to these latent conditions in the first place? There are many reasons, including the tendency of healthcare staff to seek 'shortcuts' for perceived benefits including saving time, reducing distraction and improving efficiency. Surprisingly, a tendency to migrate towards working in ways that we know to be wrong often persists. This behaviour becomes incorporated into the system and inevitably degenerates into a culture, causing claims that 'this is how we do it here' to develop.

Safe Culture and Safe Patients

Patient safety has become one of the top priorities of healthcare management. This is primarily due to emerging data from: research on patients' injuries and drug errors; cost pressures; parallel advancements in other high-risk professions; improvements in the quality of care; and changing consumer expectations. Patient safety, simplified as 'freedom from accidental injuries' from a patient perspective, is only possible in a safe environment. The safe culture of an organisation reflects individual and group values, attitudes, perceptions and competencies.

There are organisational and human factors which can affect patient safety, as stipulated in the WHO Patient Safety Methods and Measures Group report (3). The term 'human factors' is defined by UK industrial safety regulations as:

> Environmental, organisational and job factors, and human and individual characteristics, which influence behaviour at work in a way which can affect health and safety. A simple way to view human factors is to think about three aspects: the job, the individual and the organisation and how they impact on people's health-and-safety-related behaviour. (14)

In order to promote and achieve a safe culture, several changes are needed at different levels in the Swiss cheese model: the organisational and the individual levels.

Organisational level

In order to achieve and promote safe clinical practice, boardroom decisions in an organisation aimed at improving patient safety should be translated to the patient's bedside. A highly visible commitment from strong leaders is required to achieve this. The perception of effective leadership is clearly linked to lower rates of complaints from patients and better clinical governance (4). Similarly, a systematic approach should be adopted in addressing unsafe clinical practice. Dekker described the shifting foci of error investigations in a system, and a more systematic approach has subsequently been adopted into practice over the last two decades, albeit inconsistently (5). A framework described as the Human Factors Analysis and Classification System (HFACS), originally developed for use in the United States Navy and Marine Corps, could form the basis for measuring human errors (6).

HFACS describes human errors at four levels: 1) an unsafe act of the operator; 2) the preconditions for an unsafe act; 3) unsafe supervision; and 4) organisational influence. This in-depth analytical approach is designed to clarify the reasons why the error occurred in the first place. Further modifications of this approach referred to as the Human Factors Analysis and Classification System–Mining Industry Framework (HFACS-MI) is shown in Figure 9.2.

Organisational commitment to an open culture is important for a safe and error-free environment and essential for frontline staff to feel comfortable discussing patient safety issues. A safe culture should, therefore, encourage the reporting of errors and provide a just platform for learning from mistakes.

A system which operates at almost maximum capacity has been shown to migrate towards a higher risk of accidents (7). An indispensable prerequisite is adequate organisational commitment, as this would ensure effective information flow and communication to influence and improve decision making. It is interesting to note that communication failures are the leading causes of patient harm, and pre-task briefings such as WHO Surgical Safety Checklists have therefore been implemented to effectively remedy this (8). Similarly, in the armed forces, SBAR (situation, background, assessment, recommendation) is being used as an alternative communication tool (9). SBAR is an excellent method for summarising a problem. It consists of providing background information, an assessment of the situation and clear recommendations. An added advantage of this is the ability to use a common template for communication. Furthermore, changes must be 'patient centred' as evidence clearly shows that this rationale is far superior when considering patient safety.

Individual level

Discussions about the clinical care pathways of patients, including critical incidents and interventions, are routine at morbidity and mortality meetings at the clinical units of most surgical specialities. This exercise usually acts as a learning point for many practising physicians. These local meetings should act as 'error proofing' exercises and ideally be linked to a national database. On an individual or team level, various factors such as mental pressure, distractions, physical environment, physical demands, teamwork and process redesigning have been identified as foci for improvement, i.e., in view of minimising medical errors.

Is There Evidence that Simulation Training Improves Patient Safety?

Simulation is certainly not something new and has been used for millennia to, for example, plan and reduce risk, and even improve performance through hunting rituals, wedding rehearsals and mock battles. Simulation techniques for training have been successfully implemented in other professions such as sports training, the military, power generation and aviation. In the aviation industry, changes to the system without the need of additional resources brought down the accident rate from 1.19/million departures to 0.69/million departures in just one decade. This led to a successful mandatory crew resource management (CRM) training programme in the aviation industry for commercial pilots worldwide. CRM training encompasses a range of skills including situational awareness, problem solving, decision making and teamwork. In CRM training, errors are dealt with by initially reducing their rate, but if errors are to happen, early detection is promptly implemented which allows remedial action to be taken at a stage where harm is avoidable or minimised.

The penultimate question remains however: is it feasible to reliably assess the competency of human beings in terms of not making errors (safe clinical practice)? This is a difficult question to answer and no quantifiable judgement is possible. Nonetheless, in certain conditions such as stress or excessive workload, errors are more likely to take place. Scientific evidence from aviation and military research supports the inference that simulation training in the areas covered by CRM actually translates into safer flights. Similar strategies in other industry-related areas support simulation training as a means of reducing human-factor-related errors.

Simulation in Healthcare

Skills can be defined as 'action (and reaction) which an individual performs in a competent way in order to achieve a goal' (10). The prominent and important factor which separates 'novice' from 'expert' is the amount of deliberate practice carried out over a long period of time. Medical education and training faces a unique challenge as deliberate practice on a human being is becoming less possible, especially when considering diversity and variability. This, in combination with the achievements in safety in other industrial fields, has enhanced interest in simulation-based medical training. Demand is fast increasing as new healthcare technologies and delivery methods are emerging. Moreover, the demands of consumers, ethical issues and the expectations of the public are high. It has, therefore, been concluded that it is paramount that we separate training and education from the provision of actual patient care. Simulated/standardised patients have been used for objective structured clinical examinations (OSCEs) of undergraduate medical students in most medical schools across the UK. Alternative methods, such as organ models, animals and cadavers have been used in a wide array of surgical skills teaching. With the introduction of computer-based technologies, virtual reality simulation has been adopted into many surgical curricula (11). Simulators most certainly have the edge as they do not get stressed or embarrassed and their behaviour is far more predictable than that of ordinary patients. Moreover, experience and technique can be standardised to ensure reproducibility. The condition, environment and complications can be programmed using simulation technology which otherwise would need a large numbers of patients.

The shift from bedside teaching to a simulation room can also be time saving. The identification of a suitable patient, locating their investigations and potential disturbances in the busy workflow of the wards are easily avoided by the use of simulation.

The success of incorporating simulation into medical education depends on how it gets integrated into the curricula and how it becomes an essential component of lifelong learning. The quality of the skills acquired during training on simulators depends on deliberate practice that includes 'informative feedback and opportunities for repetition and correction of errors' (12). This is essential, especially when considered through the analogy that the number of years someone plays a sport or practises a profession has little impact on their quality of performance in a competition.

Competency Assessment Using Simulation

Assessment of competency using simulation-based training can be carried out using the pyramid model described by Miller (13). The levels are: a) knowledge – recall of basic facts, principles and theories; b) application of knowledge – ability to solve problems, make decisions and describe procedures; c) proof of performance – demonstrate skills in a controlled setting; and, d) action/behaviour in real practice. The method of assessment depends on the level of the learner. As they are able to recognise errors committed and suggest improvements, simulation techniques are best suited to assess all levels of competency. Using validated tools and simulators, a high degree of reliability can be attained. By minimising the variability inherent to actual clinical encounters, simulators enhance reproducibility, a fact which becomes critical when high-stake decisions depend on these assessments.

Although reported evidence of validity (face, construct or content) exists for various simulators, further research is needed in areas such as 'predictive validity'. Also, data on clinical outcomes is needed to link the simulation-based training benefits to improvement in clinical practice.

The basic objective of simulation-based skills training is to reduce the rate of medical errors and improve patient safety. This should be based on the basic educational principle of 'learning from your mistakes'. Errors have to be terminated immediately in patient-based training for their safety, however they can be allowed to progress in simulators for teaching purposes and the opportunity to rectify these does exist. Mistakes can be discussed in a simulated environment and reviewed without liability, blame or guilt. Debriefing, an essential component of simulation-based education, provides an opportunity for health professionals to improve quality of care by the innovation and implementation of new, alternative ways to manage difficult and challenging situations. Moreover, this may break the culture of silence and denial in clinical practice and improve reporting of critical incidents in a non-judgemental and productive way.

Cost-Effectiveness of Simulation in Healthcare

Assessments of cost-effectiveness, based on the reliable economic modelling of simulation-based training, have yet to be reported in literature. This needs to be addressed, as arguments can be made for and against the incorporation of technology in medical training. Whether the diversion of trainees away from the clinical environment has huge consequences for service delivery or reduces large error-based costs for the healthcare organisation is an important question that requires further research, and the last word has yet to be said on this matter.

Further research is needed to assess both the real benefits of expending resources on simulation education and its impact on the performance of healthcare professionals and healthcare organisations. It is worth mentioning here that there are some barriers to the adoption of simulation-based education. Reliable and convincing evidence in changing clinical practice is lacking, trainers often lack confidence in using simulation technology, it has high capital costs and the lack of long-term data on its impact on error reduction are just some of the more challenging issues. Nevertheless, simulation-based education seems to be a viable solution in an era of European Working Time Directives and other constraints on training in European countries in general, and the United Kingdom in particular.

Figures and Tables

Figure 8.1. The 'Swiss cheese model' of human errors

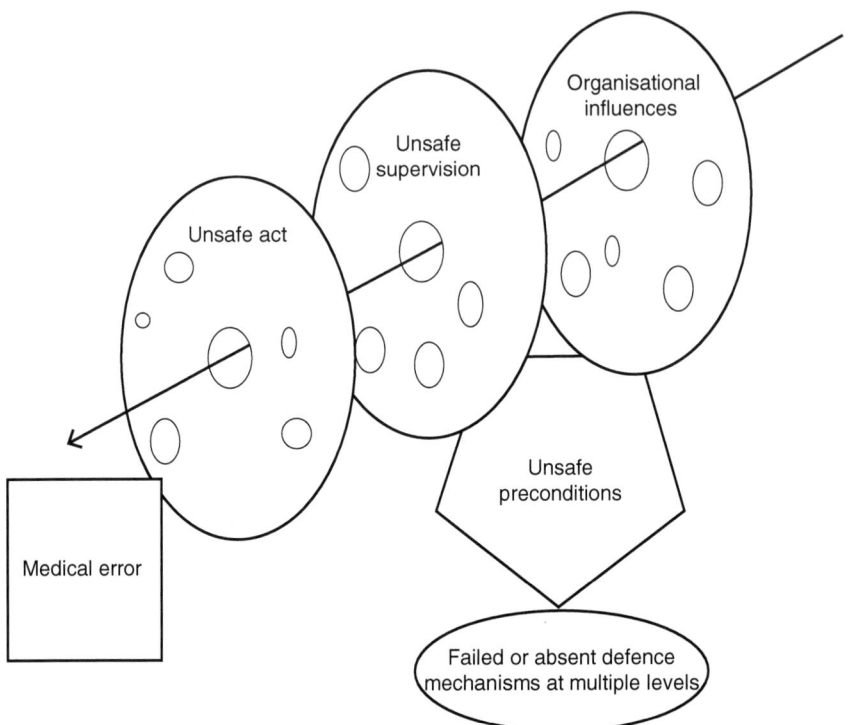

Adapted from 15.

Figure 8.2. The Human Factors Analysis and Classification System–Mining Industry Framework

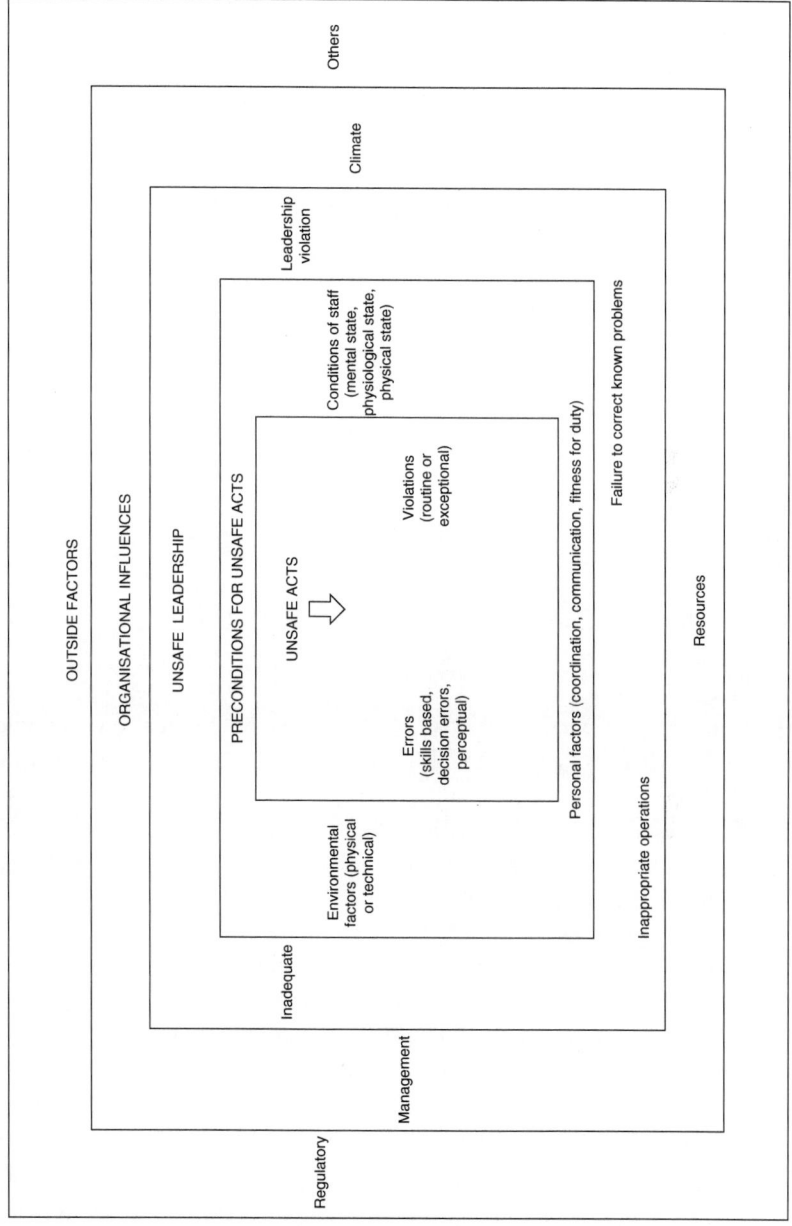

Adapted from HFACS-MI Framework report (6).

References

1. Kohn LT, Corrigan J. *To Err Is Human: Building a Safer Health System.* Washington, DC: National Academy of Sciences; 1999.
2. Barrett J, Hodgson J. Hospital simulated patient programme: a guide. *Clin Teach.* 2011;8(4):217–221.
3. Jeffs L, Law M, Michel P, Baker R. Patient safety methods and measures in acute care settings. Geneva: World Health Organization; 2009.
4. Shipton H, Armstrong C, West M, Dawson J. The impact of leadership and quality climate on hospital performance. *Int J Qual Health Care.* 2008;20(6):439–445.
5. Dekker SW. Criminalization of medical error: who draws the line? *ANZ J Surg.* 2007;77(10):831–837.
6. Shappell SA, Wiegmann DA. *The Human Factors Analysis and Classification System: The Human Factors Analysis and Classification System.* Aldershot: Ashgate; 2003.
7. Cook R, Rasmussen J. 'Going solid': a model of system dynamics and consequences for patient safety. *Qual Saf Health Care.* 2005;14(2):130–134.
8. Leonard M, Graham S, Bonacum D. The human factor: the critical importance of effective teamwork and communication in providing safe care. *Qual Saf Health Care.* 2004;13:suppl. 1:i85–90.
9. Haig KM, Sutton S, Whittington J. SBAR: a shared mental model for improving communication between clinicians. *Jt Comm J Qual Patient Saf.* 2006;32(3):167–175.
10. Issenberg SB, McGaghie WC, Hart IR, et al. Simulation technology for health care professional skills training and assessment. *JAMA.* 1999;282(9):861–866.
11. McGaghie WC, Issenberg SB, Cohen ER, Barsuk JH, Wayne DB. Does simulation-based medical education with deliberate practice yield better results than traditional clinical education? A meta-analytic comparative review of the evidence. *Acad Med.* 2011;86(6):706–711.
12. Ericsson KA. The acquisition of expert performance: an introduction to some of the issues. In: Ericsson KA. *The Road To Excellence: The Acquisition of Expert Performance in the Arts and Sciences, Sports, and Games.* Marwah, NJ: Lawrence Erlbaum Associates; 1996;1–50.
13. Miller GE. The assessment of clinical skills/competence/performance. *Acad Med.* 1990;65(9):S63–S67.
14. WHO. *Human Factors in Patient Safety Review of Topics and Tools.* World Health Organization; 2009. http://www.who.int/patientsafety/research/methods_measures/human_factors/human_factors_review.pdf. Accessed 16 December 2013.
15. Reason J. *Human Error.* Cambridge: Cambridge University Press; 1990.

Chapter 9

PSYCHOMETRICS

Jean S. Ker and Hettie Till

Chapter Objectives

This chapter will enable the reader to:

- Recognise definitions of the psychometric properties of simulation-based training;
- Analyse the psychometric properties of simulation-based assessment in differentiating trainees' performances;
- Understand how to measure the reliability of an assessment process.

Five Key Messages

1. There are a wide variety of assessment tools used to assess surgeons using simulation which can collectively provide evidence of both technical and non- technical capabilities.
2. Simulation can provide robust evidence of the level of surgical performance which is reliable and valid.
3. Psychometric analyses can be used to reliably identify those trainees who need targeted support and those who can be fast tracked through training.
4. There is emerging evidence of the validity and reliability of simulators to provide robust feedback on surgical performance.
5. The use of psychometric analyses can identify how an assessment method can be enhanced.

Introduction

The advent of new surgical techniques has brought new challenges for education and training as well as for the assessment and revalidation of surgeons (1–3). These challenges must be set against the backdrop of changing patterns of service delivery, the implementation of evidence-based practice and the increasing expectations of the public in relation to professional evidence and the accountability of competence (4). For the surgical specialties, the reduction in training time and postgraduate specialty training recommendations have halved the surgical case-load that trainees are exposed to (5). For a craft specialty, such changes can have a profound impact on the level of technical proficiency of surgeons and, ultimately, on patient safety unless appropriate interventions are introduced.

The evidence base for surgical competence comes from the use of a number of assessment tools which, when viewed together over time, can provide a profile of both the level of technical expertise as well as the non-technical capabilities of the trainee surgeon (use of NOTECHS or non-technical skills) (6–8). The use of evidence-based tools like surgical briefings has reduced the incidence of adverse events in the workplace while also setting explicit standards of surgical performance/competence (9). However, appropriate educational interventions are required to sustain these improvements and provide additional training opportunities. Simulation is one of the key initiatives that has emerged which can increase the level of technical proficiency of trainee surgeons in preparation for effective clinical practice in order to reduce the incidence of adverse events (10, 11). Simulation can also provide a safe environment for both technical and non-technical training (8, 12, 13). It enables trainees to learn in a safe environment where they can make mistakes, learn from their mistakes and also learn how to handle their mistakes without harm to themselves or to patients. In addition, simulation has a significant role to play in the prevention of skill decay.

In relation to licensing a surgeon to practise, simulation is increasingly providing evidence of the standards of practice expected (12, 14). It offers the opportunity to assess trainees at the workplace level (at the top of Miller's pyramid) (15). We can assess performance in a simulated healthcare environment at a level that the trainees should reach to practise surgery independently. The added value of using simulation is that as the focus is entirely on the learner, it is possible to assess the trainee without compromising the patient. However, like all assessment methods, the use of simulation has limitations. For instance, high-fidelity patient simulators have been used in relation to some surgical specialty training as a way of assessing both cognitive and technical competence, but published evidence on test construction, standards of instrument piloting, rater training and measures of validity and reliability is sporadic (16, 17). Indeed, there are several instances and reports which use assessment instruments to assess surgeons which have both poor validity and reliability.

There are four key questions in which psychometrics can inform the robustness of judgements made about a surgeon's professional clinical performance in a simulated setting:

1. How do we know that the assessment using simulation which we developed is good enough for the purpose that we designed it for?
2. Is the assessment using simulation effective in identifying those trainees that are competent and those who still need more practise?
3. Is the outcome a fair evaluation of the abilities of our trainees?
4. Does the assessment using simulation provide us with information about the strengths and weaknesses of our trainees in the environment in which they will have to function?

To answer these questions this chapter reviews the different psychometric properties of simulation-based assessments and demonstrates their application in practice through examples.

Psychometric Properties of Simulation-Based Assessment

All assessments must have utility (be useful). Schuwirth and Van der Vleuten produced a utility index which can serve as a framework not only for the design of assessments, but also for their evaluation (18):

$$\text{Utility} = (R - \text{reliability}) \times (V - \text{validity}) \times (A - \text{acceptability}) \\ \times (E - \text{educational impact}) \times (C - \text{cost-effectiveness}) \\ \times (P - \text{practicability})$$

Reliability: This explores whether the results of the assessment of the trainee can be reproduced and trusted.
Validity: This property focuses on whether the assessment is measuring what it is supposed to measure.
Acceptability: This component ensures that all involved in the assessment find the process appropriate.
Educational impact: This focuses on how the assessment using simulation will drive the trainee towards educationally and professionally valuable training.

Cost-effectiveness: This component explores the logistics of the assessment in terms of expenditure (money, time and manpower) in relation to the improvement in the trainee's professional performance as well as the information gained about their level of competence.

Practicability: This concentrates on the practical aspects of running and sustaining the assessment using simulation.

This utility model was endorsed by Moorthy et al. when they reviewed the current available methods of assessment of technical skills in surgery (6). In order to be useful, an assessment method must have both validity and reliability.

(1) Reliability

It is essential that we are able to provide consistent measures as evidence of the progress of trainees using simulation exercises or simulators. Reliability indicates the consistency of a measure, and an assessment instrument is said to have high reliability if it produces consistent results under consistent conditions. Error is unavoidable in any assessment and reliability is a way of describing the random error of the instrument (19). Reliability involves quantifying the consistencies of examinees' scores over different replications of the measurement procedure even though actual full replication of every measurement procedure is not necessary. Psychometric models are designed to estimate reliability through the use of different theoretical approaches or theories which include classical test theory, generalisability theory, item response theory and the multi-faceted Rasch model (MFRM).

Classical test theory

In classical test theory (CTT) we start from the assumption that the score that any candidate obtained in an assessment is just a sample of some larger set of scores which the candidate could have obtained under different circumstances. Each person thus has a 'true' score that is assumed to remain constant over different assessments, and this is the score that the person would have obtained if there were no errors in measurement (20). This means that an observed score on any assessment can be broken down into a part which is the true score (an unknown value) and an 'error' score which will vary according to the assessment taken:

$$(\text{Score}_{observed} = \text{Score}_{true} + \text{error}) \tag{21}$$

The goal of estimating reliability aims to determine how much of the variability in assessment scores is due to errors in measurement and how much is due to variability in true scores.

In CTT, reliability is commonly expressed as Cronbach's alpha. This value will generally increase as the inter-correlations among test items increase, and it is known as an internal consistency estimate of the reliability of test scores. Due to the inter-correlations among test items being maximised when all items measure the same construct, Cronbach's alpha is widely believed to indirectly indicate the degree to which a set of items measures a single uni-dimensional latent construct. Reliability is expressed as a value between 0 and 1 and the smaller the variance due to error, the higher the reliability.

Example from simulation

In a simulation assessment with three possible exercises, 141 candidates were each assessed by two assessors on the same six domains. The candidates were randomly assigned to one of three exercises. When all 12 possible scores were used, a reliability of 0.909 was obtained. This value decreased to 0.851 when only the six total scores of each domain were used (the scores of the two assessors for each domain added together). These values indicate that a very good level of internal consistency was achieved in the simulation assessment for this cohort of candidates.

Table 9.1 shows that for both the prescribing/written and health and safety domains the Cronbach's alpha value would increase if these domains were deleted from the assessment. The corrected item–total correlation values were also lower for these two domains, especially the health and safety one. This is an indication that these domains did not discriminate well between the candidates and would need to be reviewed before being used in subsequent simulation assessments.

Generalisability theory

According to generalisability theory (G-theory), there are many potential sources of error, suggesting that the CTT model of the observed score being the sum of two components, i.e., a true score and an error score, is too simplistic. G-theory analyses allow for multiple sources of error to be 'disentangled' and a G-theory analysis is started by trying to identify all possible sources of error (facets) that could impact on the candidate scores in that particular assessment (20). In our simulation example these would include, inter alia, different candidate abilities, different assessor severity/leniency measures, different difficulty levels of the exercises used and the fact that some of the domains are more difficult to score high marks in than others. The average score obtained over all of these facets is called a universe score and differs from the one true score of CTT. In G-theory different sets of variables (facets) will yield different universe scores.

The first part of G-theory (the G-study) is an analysis of variance (ANOVA) which estimates the variance attributed to each of the identified facets and the interactions amongst these facets, as well as the variance attributable to what is considered error. This is followed by a decision study (D-study) in which the numbers of each level of a facet can be varied and the effect of the change on the reliability (the generalizability coefficient) observed (21). Questions such as whether it might be better to use two assessors instead of one, or whether the number of items should be increased or not, can be addressed in the D-study.

Example from simulation

In the simulation assessment described above, the G-study showed an overall internal consistency (generalizability coefficient) of 0.818. The results of the G-study ANOVA is shown in Table 9.2. Assessors, tasks to be completed in the simulation exercises and other facets can influence the precision with which the candidate scores are measured. From Table 9.2 it appears as though the assessors (a : s : e) did not contribute large amounts to the variability of the observed scores. The small effect of the assessors suggests that they ranked the candidates similarly and this was supported by an inter-rater reliability of 0.895.

The main source of estimated variation (38%) came from candidates nested in exercise (c : e). This indicates that a large amount of the variance is attributable to systematic differences between the objects of measurement (candidates). The larger the percentage of variance accounted for by the candidates, the higher the reliability (21).

Candidates are randomly assigned to complete one of three possible simulation assessment exercises. Table 9.2 shows that the effect of exercise (e) is small, which indicates that there were not large differences in the levels of difficulty between simulation exercises. This is a good result as different difficulty levels between the exercises would indicate a bias in the assessment. The D-study follows the G-study and is used to explore what the overall reliability would be under various conditions. In our simulation example, CCT analyses (Table 9.1) indicated that some of our domains (items) did not discriminate well between the candidates. The G-study results (Table 9.2) indicated that some of the variance is attributable to items (i). One possibility to improve the simulation assessment would be to split domains that might measure more than one 'construct' and develop more domains to test the candidates on. In our D-study we thus explored the effect that using more items would have on the generalizability coefficient. Table 9.3 shows that increasing the number of items would increase the generalizability coefficient.

Multi-faceted Rasch model

All assessments are designed to measure a variable, or variables, of interest. Depending on the type of assessment, these might be surgical proficiency or clinical reasoning, but these abilities, or traits, are unobservable, or latent. The main goal of designing assessments that are 'fit for purpose' is to try to measure how much of a latent trait a trainee possesses. Traits cannot be measured directly and we usually have to rely on the expert judgement of assessors to provide the trainee with a set of scores. Most clinical assessments, including those involving simulation, rely on assessors judging trainee performances in a complex environment in which there are many variables that can impact on the trainees' performance and, thus, on their ability scores. As with the G-study discussed above, the MFRM analyses include variables (facets) that impact on the candidates' scores in terms of candidate ability, assessor severity/leniency measures, item (domain) difficulty and so on. Performance assessments, such as simulation assessments, often involve the judging of candidates by a number of assessors over a number of sessions. Provided the judging plan creates a linking network with, for example, assessors judging more than one session in the same domains, it is possible to calculate estimates of candidate ability, examiner severity, item difficulty or any other facet included that could all be reported on one common linear scale (22). Using this approach allows one to look at the various facets and draw useful comparisons between them.

Example from simulation

In a simulation assessment 16 candidates were each assessed by three assessors on the same seven domains. From a three-facet Rasch model, a vertical ruler (Figure 9.1) was obtained indicating candidate performance as well as assessor severity/leniency and item (domain) difficulty on the same logit (log-odds) scale. From Figure 9.1 it can be seen that this assessment discriminated well between the candidates. The column headed '+Candidates' shows the candidate spread from most able at the top (3.04 logits) to least able at the bottom (−3.18 logits), a range of 6.2 logits. This exam was able to reliably (.95) separate the candidates into about six levels of ability.

The vertical ruler shows the assessor spread from most severe at the top (1.58 logits) to most lenient at the bottom (−1.47 logits) in the column headed 'Assessors'. Figure 9.1 also indicates that the different domains had different levels of difficulty. It was most difficult to score high marks in the prescribing/written domain and easiest in the response to interruptions. The Rasch measures accounted for 56.86% of the total variance in the ratings, of which the variance explained by the candidates was 39.0%, by the assessors, 7.2%, and by the domains, 10.7%. Even though this simulation exercise was taken by a different group of candidates from the one described in the CTT and G-theory examples above, they were tested on the same domains. From this MFRM analysis it again becomes apparent that some of the variability in candidate scores (10.7%) is attributable to the domain factor. This result supported our decision to improve the simulation assessment by splitting those domains that might measure more than one 'construct' and developing more domains to test the candidates on.

In an MFRM analysis the Facets computer program adjusts candidate ability measures for differences in the level of severity/leniency that individual assessors exercise. Since different sets of assessors usually rate each candidate, some candidates may have been unfairly advantaged if they happened to be rated by more lenient assessors, while other candidates may have been unfairly disadvantaged if they happened to be rated by more severe assessors. For each candidate, Facets calculates a 'fair average' measure which indicates the candidate's level of ability that assessors of average severity/leniency would have rated that candidate (23).

(2) Validity

Any simulation-based assessment involving the development of technical skills and non-technical skills needs to be relevant to the developing expertise of the trainee. Clinical assessments are not valid or invalid: it is only a matter of degree. The term 'validity' refers to whether the assessment is actually measuring the performance or competence it was designed to measure. There have been a number of reports and studies in academic literature relating to the validity of surgical simulators as tools for assessing technical skills, and there is an emerging literature relating to the valid assessment of non-technical skills and performance in a simulated healthcare context (8, 24–27).

There are a number of types of validity, such as content validity, face validity, construct validity, concurrent validity and predictive validity. Their definitions in surgical literature are not consistent but include terms linked to direct or indirect validity categories.

Content validity

This is the extent to which a domain that is being assessed in a simulated exercise is being adequately sampled. For example, in surgery this may link to knot tying in different scenarios using laparoscopic techniques. In relation to a more immersive simulation in a healthcare context, this may refer to the adequate sampling of patient presentations to assess surgeons' diagnostic skills at a level commensurate with standards expected. This often involves developing a blueprint for assessment aligned to a curricular programme. The length of each simulation scenario should reflect the skill being assessed with adequate sampling of skills in different contexts.

Face validity

This is the extent to which the simulation or simulator appears to reflect real clinical experience. In a surgical context this may be seen in the use of animal materials in the development of technical skills or a virtual reality simulator which can recreate the technical and environmental aspects of surgical practice.

Construct validity

A construct is a personal psychological characteristic that cannot be observed directly. For example, in surgery one would expect that those who demonstrated problem solving skills in a knot tying simulation exercise using animal material would demonstrate the same capability of problem solving in a virtual surgical simulator.

Predictive validity

This aspect of validity relates to whether an assessment can predict performance at a later stage. For example, performance in a simulated assessment exercise in surgery will correlate to future performance in the workplace. Looking at this in another way, one would expect an expert surgeon to perform better according to the assessment criteria in a simulated exercise than a novice surgical trainee would.

(3) Acceptability

Some of the major challenges of using simulation in performance assessment include ensuring that the exercises/tasks used to assess trainees are aligned to those required to function in the workplace and ascertaining that everyone involved in the assessment finds the process appropriate. In relation to developing a simulation exercise for assessment, acceptability can be enhanced through developing an online orientation PowerPoint presentation which describes where manikins or simulated patients will be used. Ensuring the physical fidelity of, for example, a surgical ward or theatre will enable trainee surgeons to immerse themselves in an environment similar to the workplace. This should incorporate interruptions as well as the sounds and smells evocative of practice (27).

Another way of ensuring that trainees and assessors find the simulation assessment acceptable is to require them to complete an evaluation questionnaire concerning its realism at the end of the simulated assessment exercise.

(4) Cost-Effectiveness

This component focuses on the logistics of the assessment in terms of its expenditure (money, time and manpower) in relation to the improvement of the trainee's professional performance, as well as the information that is gained about the trainee's level of competence. The clarity of what is being assessed and how it is being assessed contributes to judgements about the cost-effectiveness of an assessment exercise.

Example of cost-effectiveness in a simulation

If simulation is to be used to assess performance in the workplace then aspects of the workplace have to be recreated in the simulation-based assessment. However, engagement in a simulation assessment can be established with minimal resources through the introduction of relevant cues like time pressures. This can contribute to reliably informing judgements made on a trainee's clinical performance in the simulated setting. The development of such exercises must be meticulous and conscious of detail and can therefore initially be time-consuming and costly in terms of set-up costs. Ongoing operating costs for consumables and the organisation associated with running the assessment can also be high. A degree of forward planning concerning the number of assessors required and development of a training programme should also be incorporated into the whole process, considering time, expertise and a backfill of personnel. In addition, the training of simulated patients and the preparation of manikins and specialist equipment to develop pre-determined scenarios need to be considered as part of the overall business case. This ensures that the standards of simulation-based scenarios are maintained and their quality assures the outcome of the assessment process. The advantages of having trainees learn, make mistakes and then learn from their mistakes in a safe environment without compromising patients enhances their self-assessment, making the use of simulation in the assessment of performance a worthwhile and cost-effective endeavour.

(5) Educational Impact

Any assessment process and its outcome has an impact on how trainees prepare themselves and behave in their professional role in the workplace; i.e., whether they focus more on the acquisition of knowledge or on the application of knowledge in relation to their professional practice. In surgery this could relate to the safe practice of both technical and non-technical skills, for example knot tying or the use of the surgical pause developed as a patient safety tool for operating theatres. The educational impact of any assessment relates to both the process of the assessment and its outcome, or how it drives the trainees towards appropriate educational and professional training. In addition, the rating method used in an assessment such as a Likert-type scale or a binary checklist can impact on how trainees learn or memorise the steps used in a procedure. The use of rating scales tends to encourage expert judgements and a more holistic approach which can focus the assessment onto higher cognitive levels by ensuring the application of required skills in different situations.

Example from simulation

Ward simulation exercises use rating scales to judge the capability of trainees according to the standards of the GMC's Good Medical Practice during their performance in a simulated work shift (27).

(6) Practicability

This focuses on the practical aspects of running and sustaining the assessment using simulation. The trend of using portfolio assessment with sampling assessment of areas of practice over time presents a unique opportunity to develop a profile of evidence concerning practice. Simulation offers a practical opportunity to provide video evidence of performance that can be reliably compared between the trainees without compromising safe patient care.

Summary

Psychometrically sound assessment using simulation enables evidence of surgeons' performance to be presented objectively and with a robustness which reassures one that standards of operative practice are in place for each surgeon and that these represent a fair evaluation of their capabilities.

The use of psychometric analyses from a simulated assessment can also provide information on the strengths and weaknesses of surgeons' performance.

Given that morbidity and mortality data only provide a limited picture of a surgeon's capability, it is the evidence from these different assessments which can identify performance issues, highlighting where support needs to be targeted and where trainees can be accelerated through training using the most effective and efficient simulator or simulation event.

Tables and Figures

Table 9.1. Item-total statistics of the domain total scores

Domain	Scale mean if item deleted	Scale variance if item deleted	Corrected item–total correlation	Cronbach's alpha if item deleted
Clinical skills	33.99	38.550	0.790	0.798
Critically ill patient	34.27	38.084	0.719	0.809
Prescribing/ written	34.05	43.162	0.493	0.852
Response to interruptions	33.53	40.451	0.733	0.810
Communication	33.24	39.227	0.702	0.813
Health and safety	33.96	43.377	0.427	0.867

Table 9.2. Results of G-study ANOVA showing estimates of variance components

Source	Degrees of freedom	Sum of squares	Mean squares	Variance component
e	2	21.12194	10.56097	0.00910
c : e	138	639.17356	4.63169	0.31168
a : c : e	141	52.33333	0.37116	0.03333
i	5	50.82033	10.16407	0.03068
ei	10	15.04415	1.50442	0.00868
ci : e	690	477.13552	0.69150	0.26017
ai : c : e	705	120.66667	0.17116	0.17116

e = exercise; c = candidate; a = assessor; i = item

Table 9.3. Results of D-study changing number of items only

Number of items	Generalizability coefficient
6	0.818
7	0.837
8	0.852
9	0.864
10	0.873
11	0.982

Figure 9.1. Variable map comparing marks on a common logit scale for candidate ability, assessor stringency, item (domain) difficulty and scaled marks

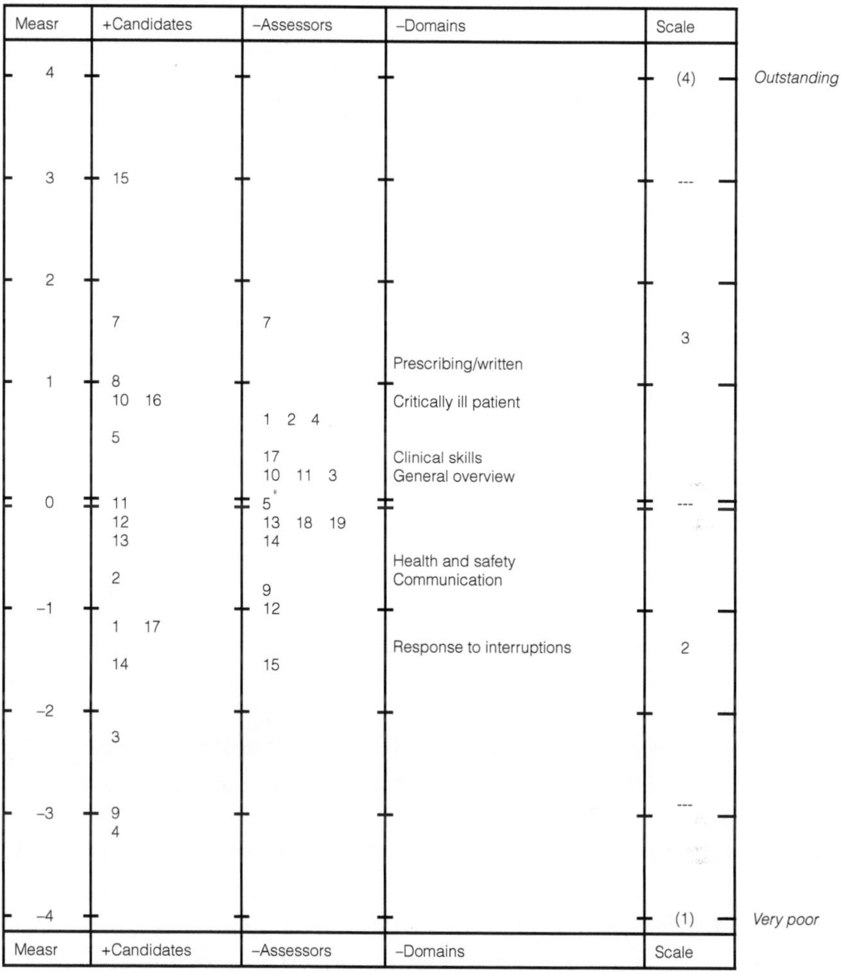

Measr	+Candidates	−Assessors	−Domains	Scale	
4				(4)	Outstanding
3	15			---	
2					
	7	7		3	
1	8		Prescribing/written		
	10 16	1 2 4	Critically ill patient		
	5	17	Clinical skills		
		10 11 3	General overview		
0	11	5		---	
	12	13 18 19			
	13	14	Health and safety		
	2	9	Communication		
−1	1 17	12			
	14	15	Response to interruptions	2	
−2	3				
−3	9			---	
	4				
−4				(1)	Very poor
Measr	+Candidates	−Assessors	−Domains	Scale	

References

1. Fairhurst K, Strickland A, Maddern G. Simulation speak. *Journal of Surgical Education*. 2011;68(5):382–386.
2. Cuschieri A, Francis N, Crosby J, Hanna GB. What do master surgeons think of surgical competence and revalidation? *Am J Surg*. 2001;182: 110–116.
3. Reznik R, Reghr G, MacCrae H, Martin J, McCulloch W. Testing technical skill via an innovative bench station examination. *Am J Surg*. 1997;173:226–230.
4. Darzi A, Smith S, Taffinder N. Assessing operative skill needs to become more objective. *BMJ*. 1999;318:887–888.
5. Leach D. A model for GME: shifting from process to outcomes. A progress report from the Accreditation Council for Graduate Medical Education. *Med Ed*. 2004;38:4–12.
6. Moorthy K, Munz Y, Sarkar S, Darzi A. Objective assessment of technical skills in surgery. *BMJ*. 2003;327:1032–1037.
7. Reznick R, MacCrae H. Teaching surgical skills: changes in the wind. *NEJM*. 2011;355(25):2664–2669.
8. McCulloch P, Mishra A, Handa A, Dale T, Hirst G, Catchpole K. The effects of aviation-style non-technical skills on technical performance and outcome in the operating theatre. *Qual Saf in Healthcare*. 2009;18:109–115.
9. Lingard L, Regehr G, Orser B, et al. Evaluation of a pre-operative checklist and team briefing amongst surgeons, nurses and anaesthesiologists to reduce failures in communication. *Arch Surg*. 2008;143(1):12–17.
10. Strom P, Kjellin A, Hedman L. Validation and learning in the procedures KSA virtual reality surgical simulator. *Surg Endosc*. 2003;17:227–231.
11. Gauger P, Hauge LS, Andreatta P, et al. Laparoscopic simulation training with proficiency targets improves practice and performance of novice surgeons. *Am J Surg*. 2010(199):72–80.
12. Freid GM, Feldman LS, Vassilou MC, et al. Proving the value of simulation in laparoscopic surgery. *Ann Surg*. 2004;240(3):518–528.
13. Moorthy K, Munz Y, Forrest D, Pandey V, Undre S, Vincent C. Surgical crisis management skills training and assessment: a simulation-based approach to enhancing operating room performance. *Ann Surg*. 2006;244(1):139–147.
14. Seymour NE. VR or OR: a review of evidence that virtual reality simulation improves operating room performance. *World J Surg*. 2008;32:182–188.
15. Miller G. The assessment of clinical skills/competence/performance. *Acad Med*. 1990;65:S63–S67.

16. Edler AA, Fanning R, Chen M, et al. Patient simulation: a literary synthesis of assessment tools in anaesthesiology. *Journal of Educational Evaluation for Healthcare Professionals*. 2009;6:1–9.
17. Boulet JR, Murray D, Woodhouse J, McAllister J, Ziv A. Reliability and validity of a simulation-based acute care skills assessment for medical students and residents. *Anaesthesiology*. 2003;99(6):1270–1280.
18. Schuwirth LWT, Van der Vleuten CPM. How to design a useful test: the principles of assessment. In: Swanwick T, ed. *Understanding Medical Education, Evidence, Theory and Practice*. 2nd ed. Oxford: Wiley-Blackwell; 2013:243–255.
19. Brennan RL, ed. *Educational Measurement*, fourth edition. Westport, CT: Preager; 2006.
20. Brennan RL. Performance assessments from the perspective of generalizability theory. *Applied Psychological Measurement*. 2000;24(4):339–353.
21. Streiner DL, Norman GR. *Health Measurement Scales: A Practical Guide to Their Development and Use*, fourth edition. New York: Oxford University Press; 2008.
22. Linacre JM, Wright BD. Construction of measures from many-facet data. *Journal of Applied Measurement*. 2002;3(4):484–509.
23. Linacre JM. Communicating examinee measures as expected ratings. *Rasch Measurement Transactions*. 1997;11(1):550–551. http://www.rasch.org/rmt/rmt111m.htm. Accessed 12 December 2013.
24. Paisley AM, Baldwin PJ, Paterson-Brown S. Validity of surgical simulation for the assessment of operative skills. *Br J of Surg*. 2001;88:1525–1532.
25. Scott DJ, Bergen PC, Rege RV. Laparoscopic training on bench models: better and more cost-effective than operating room experience? *J Am Coll Surg*. 2000;191:272–283.
26. Gallagher AG, Ritter EM, Champion H, et al. Virtual reality simulation for the operating room: proficiency-based training as a paradigm shift in surgical skills training. *Ann Surg*. 2005;241(2):364–372.
27. Ker JS, Hesketh EA, Anderson F, Johnstone D. Can a ward simulation exercise provide the realism required to provide evidence for full registration decisions for borderline PRHOs? The results of a feasibility study. *Medical Teacher*. 2006;28(4):330–334.

Chapter 10

FUTURE OF SURGICAL SIMULATION

Iain S. Tait and Benjie Tang

Current Developments in Simulation Models for Surgical Skills Training

In 1892, Professor William Halsted introduced the first apprenticeship system for surgical training at Johns Hopkins Hospital, Baltimore. The modernisation of medical careers and shorter training programmes have challenged this traditional approach, and in recent years surgical education and training have developed into a curriculum-based system to ensure that students acquire core skills to gain a basic proficiency in surgery (1). Advances in medical technology, the evolution of laparoscopic surgery and the introduction of Working Time Directives have dictated changes to the system of surgical training and identified an increased need for the safe, controlled practice of simulation and simulators that are specific to surgical training (1–4).

Learning by procedure-based simulators has definite advantages over performing operative procedures and practising on patients (Figures 10.1–10.3) (5). Simulation enables the surgical trainee to acquire essential skills and progress along a proficiency curve before attempting a real procedure, and provides them with a low-risk environment in which to rehearse and practise their technique without stress or tight time constraints (1–7).

Learning by simulation models allows surgical trainees to commit errors that are an essential component of the learning process (8–11). These simulated systems are also valuable for surgical skills assessment because they enable standardised training through the repeated practice of skills and procedures under standardised conditions (12). The benefits of simulation training are now being increasingly recognised and, consequently, there has been a considerable development in the role of simulators and simulation in surgical training (1–3, 5–12).

A simulation-based surgical training programme can be structured and developed to ensure the acquisition of essential surgical skills by junior surgical trainees (1, 2, 4, 13–16). Within surgical education and training, surgical skills courses for both open and laparoscopic skills at a basic level have been proven to be valid and effective means of surgical skills acquisition (1–3, 8, 17–19). Standard surgical skills can be learned and practised on synthetic, animate models and virtual reality (VR) simulators in skills training laboratories, and then transferred to the operating theatre (5, 19–21). Thus, skills are developed in a safe environment prior to embarking on surgery on real patients (11, 20).

Many surgical training courses have been developed, validated and standardised using simulation and simulators (5, 11, 19–21). For example, the Advanced Trauma Life Support (ATLS) is widely accepted as an essential basic skills course that teaches surgeons about the fundamental principles of the initial resuscitation of the multiply-injured trauma patient (22, 23).

The Simulab TraumaMan human patient simulator (HPS) and advanced HPS have been proven to be equivalent to more traditional means of teaching the course (15). TraumaMan is a life-like human torso with which students can practise chest tube insertion, pericardiocentesis, peritoneal lavage and cricothyroidotomy (22). The advanced HPS (Medical Education Technologies Inc., Sarasota, FL) allows students to practise intubation, needle thoracentesis, tube thoracostomy, peri-cardiocentesis and intravenous catheterisation. Studies have demonstrated that skills learned and acquired using simulation-based medical education for trauma improve the clinician's readiness to employ essential knowledge, skills, and abilities for acute patient care (13, 14, 22, 23).

Similarly, inexperienced surgical trainees can learn and practise surgical skills to an intermediate level and perform simulated procedures such as laparoscopic appendicectomy and laparoscopic cholecystectomy on both VR simulators and animate animal models in the training laboratory (21, 24–26).

Many studies have demonstrated that computer-based VR simulators improve the performance of laparoscopic tasks, and that skills acquired from VR simulators can be transferred to the operating room (2, 3, 15, 17, 21, 25, 27). Seymour et al. demonstrated that gallbladder dissection was 29% faster when performed by VR-trained residents while non-VR-trained residents were nine times more likely to fail to make progress. Similar benefits have been demonstrated with the LapSim VR simulator, whereby laparoscopic surgery skills are increased in a clinically relevant manner using proficiency-based virtual reality simulator training (2). Other studies have shown similar gains in skill acquisition using commercially available VR simulators (27).

Animal tissue models have also proved to be a useful simulation model for surgeons to rehearse the key steps of surgical procedures such as laparoscopic fundoplication, gastric bypass procedure, common bile duct exploration, sigmoidectomy, lung lobectomy, and nephrectomy (26, 29, 30). This approach has proven to be effective, relatively inexpensive and accurately simulates the clinical procedure (29, 30).

What is the Future of Procedure-Based Simulation?

Anaesthetised animals are suitable to use for acquiring advanced laparoscopic skills (28) and also performing specific laparoscopic procedures such as laparoscopic gastric bypass and liver surgery (28, 31). Live porcine simulation is useful for skills acquisition for the laparoscopic gastric bypass procedure, while live sheep have been identified as good models for practising laparoscopic hepatic resection (31). However, there are concerns about using live animals for surgical training as their anatomy is quite different to that of humans, and thus they do not provide an accurate simulation. There are also ethical issues around animal well-being, the logistics of course delivery and concerns for the health and safety of course participants. In some countries, including the UK, the use of live animals for surgical training is prohibited.

The human cadaver is recognised as the only truly authentic simulation model for surgical training, and is presently regarded as the most realistic non-patient model for specific surgical procedure training (32–36). Therefore, human cadavers are increasingly used for advanced courses in surgical training. Traditional formalin-fixed, Thiel-fixed (or alternative soft-fix) and fresh cadavers are all available and used for advanced surgical training.

However it is the Thiel-fixed (soft-fix) and fresh cadavers that are preferred to the formalin-embalmed bodies for surgical training, as the colour, texture and consistency of organs, the flexibility, plasticity and preservation of the tissue plane of the tissue and organs and the articulation of the joints are very similar to in vivo conditions (33, 34).

Based on the current success of using human cadavers for orthopaedic surgery and laparoscopic surgery training, and the development of the new Thiel technique for preserving human bodies in a life-like state (Figure 10.1) (32–36), surgical training courses across all surgical specialties can now be designed and developed, which was not previously possible with formalin-embalmed bodies (32–36).

Whilst soft-fix human cadavers have immense potential for use on technical skills training programmes, it is essential that these cadaveric training courses are integrated into recognised and accredited surgical training curricula which preferably include training in both technical and non-technical skills in the simulated environment (32–35).

Evidence Regarding Patient Safety

The Institute of Medicine reported that between 44,000 and 98,000 patients die from medical errors (including surgical errors) every year in the USA (37). Surgery contributes to almost 50% of recorded adverse events and up to 13% of all hospital deaths (37, 38). The Institute of Medicine reported that 100 patients die from iatrogenic injuries in US hospitals each day and that 40% of these injuries are committed in the operating room (40, 38, 39). Deficiencies in non-technical skills are repeatedly identified as important contributors to adverse events and remain a key cause of surgical errors worldwide (41–44).

Population-based studies have indicated that most adverse surgical events are preventable (39, 40, 45, 46). Therefore prescriptive error reduction or prevention systems are important in ensuring a good surgical outcome. However, error reduction systems have to be based on objective information about the nature of intraoperative technical errors, and designed to educate surgical trainees in non-technical skills (47, 48).

Future of Non-technical Skills Simulation (NOTSS)

Historically, surgical training has focused on technical skills to improve task performance and the quality of operations (49, 50). However, it is recognised that a skilfully performed operation is 75% decision-making ability and 25% technical dexterity (51). Thus the non-technical skills of situation awareness, decision making, task management, communication skills, leadership and teamwork are the critical factors that determine the quality of surgery and patient safety.

Evidence suggests that these non-technical elements can enhance a surgeon's technical performance (48). Non-technical skills training is common practice in civil aviation (52), oil exploration (53), anaesthesia (54) and nuclear power but it is only recently that non-technical skills for successful surgery have been included in the surgical curriculum (55, 56).

A number of observational-based systems have been developed to study non-technical performance in the operating room, namely Non-technical Skills for Surgeons (NOTSS) (58), NOTECHS from an earlier non-technical skills aviation instrument (57) and Observational Teamwork Assessment for Surgery (OTAS) (60). Non-technical skills are relatively procedure-independent and can thus be assessed on a wide variety of appropriate procedures using NOTSS (59). NOTECHS was originally developed for the aviation industry for crew resource management (CRM) and has been adapted for safe practice in anaesthesia (54) and surgery (47, 48, 57). OTAS was developed for the assessment of factors that are important in patient outcomes and also has the functionality to evaluate teamwork in the operating theatre (60, 61).

A systematic review of the impact of non-technical skills on technical performance in surgery highlighted that the majority of research into non-technical skills focused on communication, leadership, teamwork and decision making (47). However, it should also be recognised that: (i) a lack of situational awareness is associated with a high rate of technical errors; (ii) the ability to cope with excessive levels of stress in the operating theatre is key to maintaining optimum technical performance; (iii) increased levels of fatigue have a negative impact on surgical performance; (iv) provision of feedback has beneficial effects on certain aspects of technical performance; and, (v) the impact of communications skills on technical performance is still unclear (47, 59).

Therefore, future training in a simulated operating theatre should provide surgical trainees with an environment and facilities to practise and improve their technical and non-technical skills for: (i) routine technical procedures; and (ii) crisis scenario training, with the integration of training in both technical and non-technical skills (56, 62).

Simulated operating theatres have gradually gained acceptance for training in surgical crisis management and specific technical procedures (62–64). In simulated team training it is possible to focus on both elements, allowing trainees to practise their technical skills and also their non-technical skills of communication, situational awareness, teamwork, leadership, and decision making (Figure 10.2) (62, 63, 65).

Franc-Law and his team conducted a randomised study to compare patient flow during a simulated disaster and found that the group with simulation training triaged patients more quickly than the control group (43 versus 75 seconds, p<0.001) and scored higher in task performance (18/18 versus 8/18, p<0.001) (14). In another simulated emergency study, Marshall et al. demonstrated that training on computerised human patient simulators (HPS) in conjunction with ATLS training enhanced the clinician's trauma management skills (13).

In a further recent study investigating the value of high-fidelity simulation training, Park et al. found that event-specific, simulation-based training resulted in superior performance in scenarios compared with traditional training (66). The simulation of operating theatres and other clinical environments will play an essential role in future skills training curricula.

Summary

Several factors have contributed to the changes in surgical training that have led to some key elements of surgical skills training taking place outside the operating theatre. To facilitate this more structured curriculum-based training programme, there have been significant developments in bench-top models, synthetic physical models, restructured animal tissue models, live animal models, VR simulators and human cadavers for teaching and practising the technical elements of surgical skills training. The potential benefits and advantages of these surgical simulation models which facilitate practice in low-risk environments are widely recognised.

However, deficiencies in non-technical skills are identified as important contributors to adverse events in the clinical environment, and especially in surgery. Therefore, it is equally important that surgeons focus on their non-technical skills to improve the quality of their performance in the operating theatre. The simulated operating theatre will play a significant role in the future training of both individual surgeons and clinical teams for technical and non-technical skills.

Key Messages

1. Patient-based surgical skills practice is not desirable.
2. Synthetic tissue models, restructured animal tissue models, VR simulators and cadaveric models provide excellent simulation for surgical training.
3. The acquisition of core knowledge and key technical skills is essential.
4. Non-technical skills also impact on technical performance.
5. Simulated operating theatres enable individuals and surgical teams to learn and practise technical and non-technical skills in a low-risk environment.

Figures and Tables

Table 10.1. Proposed draft non-technical skills taxonomy

Interpersonal skills	Cognitive skills
Communication	Situation awareness
Leadership	Mental readiness
Teamwork	Assessing risks
Briefing/planning/preparation	Anticipating problems
Resource management	Decision making
Seeking advice and feedback	Adaptive strategies/flexibility
Coping with pressure/stress/fatigue	Workload distribution

FUTURE OF SURGICAL SIMULATION   117

Figure 10.1. Human cadaver preserved using a new Thiel technique for laparoscopic colorectal surgery training (Cuschieri Skills Centre, Dundee)

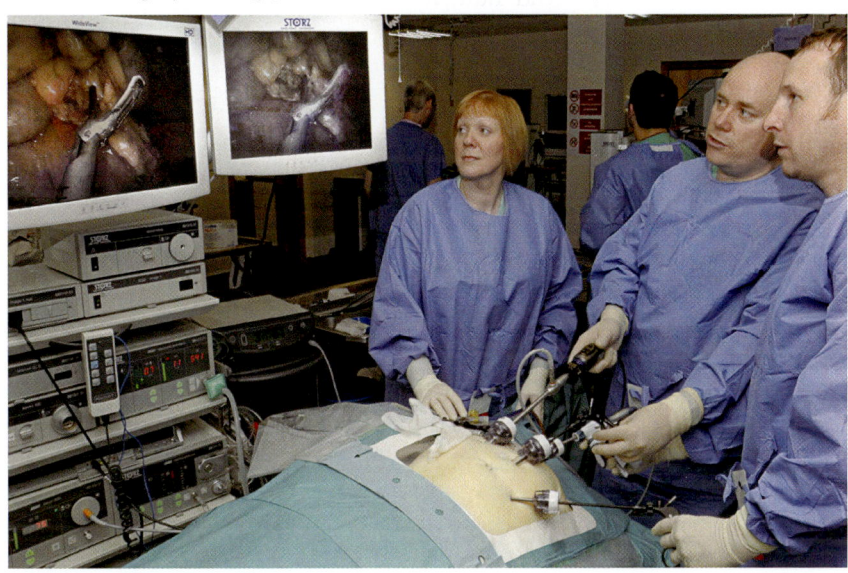

Figure 10.2. Simulated operating room for surgical team training (Cuschieri Skills Centre, Dundee)

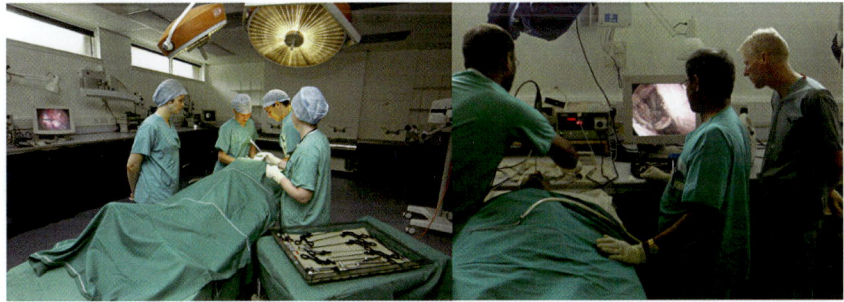

Figure 10.3. Simulation-based training for sinus surgery (Cuschieri Skills Centre, Dundee)

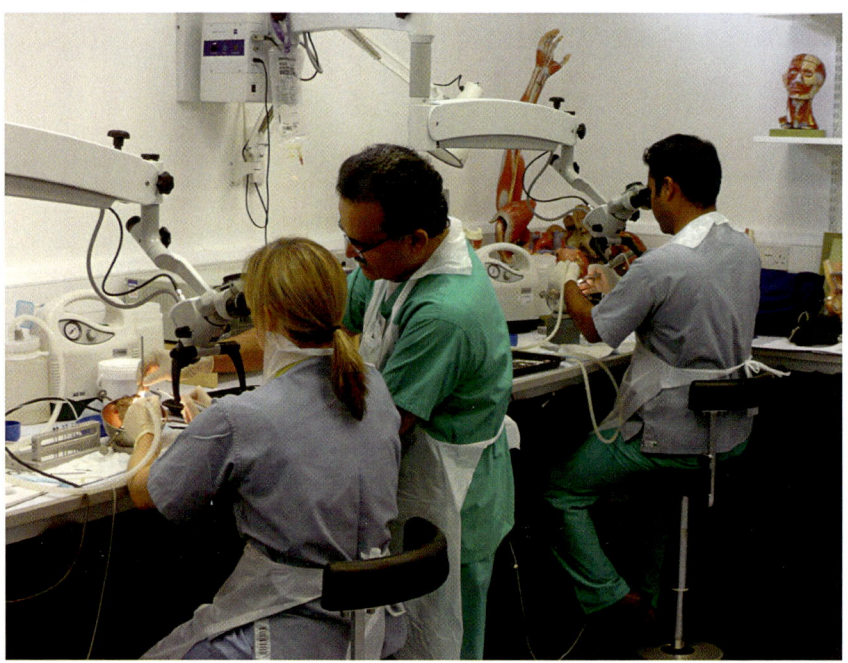

References

1. Sott DJ. Patient safety, competency, and the future of surgical simulation. *Simulation in Healthcare*. 2006;1:164–170.
2. Larsen CR, Soerensen JL, Grantcharov TP, et al. Effect of virtual reality training on laparoscopic surgery: randomized controlled trial. *BMJ*. 2009;338:b1802.
3. Schout MBA, Hendrikx AJ, Scheele F, et al. Validation and implementation of surgical simulators: a critical review of present, past, and future. *Surg Endosc*. 2010;24:536–546.
4. Giles JA. Surgical training and the European working time directive: the role of informal workplace learning. *Int J Surg*. 2010;8(3):179–80.
5. Scott DJ, Bergen PC, Rege RV, et al. Laparoscopic training on bench models: better and more cost effective than operating room experience? *J Am Coll Surg*. 2000;1919:272–283.
6. McGaghie WC, Issenberg SB, Petrusa ER, et al. A critical review of simulation-based medical education research, 2003–2009. *Med Edu*. 2010;44:50–63.

7. Gallagher AG, Ritter EM, Champion H, et al. Virtual reality simulation for the operating room: proficiency-based training as a paradigm shift in surgical skills training. *Ann Surg.* 2005;241:464–372.
8. Reznick RK, MacRae H. Teaching surgical skills: changes in the wind. *N Engl J Med.* 355:2664–2669.
9. Blumenthal D. Making medical errors into 'medical treasure'. *JAMA.* 1994;272:1867–1868.
10. Kneebone RL, Scott W, Darzi A, et al. Simulation and clinical practice: strengthening the relationship. *Med Educ.* 2004;38:1095–1102.
11. Derossis AM, Abrahamowicz M, Sigman HH, et al. Development of a model for training and evaluation of laparoscopic skills. *Am J Surg.* 1998;175:482–487.
12. Issenberg SB, McGaghie WC, Hart IR, et al. Simulation technology for healthcare professional skills training and assessment. *JAMA.* 1999;282:861–866.
13. Marshall RL, Smith JS, Corman PJ, et al. Use of human patient simulators in the development of resident trauma management skills. *Trauma.* 2001;51:17–21.
14. Franc-Law JM, Ingrassia PL, Ragazzoni L, et al. The effectiveness of training with an emergency department simulator on medical student performance in a simulated disaster. *CJEM.* 2010;12:27–32.
15. Cherry RA, Williams J, George J, et al. The effectiveness of a human patient simulator in the ATLS shock skills station. *J Surg Res.* 2007;139:229–235.
16. Cherry RA, Ali J. Current concepts in simulation-based trauma education. *Trauma.* 2008;65:1186–1193.
17. Seymour NE, Gallagher AG, Roman SA et al. Virtual reality training improves operating room performance: results of a randomized, double-blinded study. *Ann Surg.* 2002;236:458–463.
18. Mackay S, Datta V, Chang A, et al. Multiple objective measures of skills (MOMS): a new approach to the assessment of technical ability in surgical trainees. *Ann Surg.* 2003;238:291–300.
19. Aggarwal R, Grantcharov TP, Eriksen JR, et al. An evidence-based virtual reality training program for novice laparoscopic surgeons. *Ann Surg.* 2006;244:310–314.
20. Scott DJ, Dunnington GL. The new ACS/APDS skills curriculum: moving the learning curve out of the operating room. *J Gastrointest Surg.* 2008;12:213–221.
21. Sturm LP, Windsor JA, Cosman PH, et al. A systematic review of skills transfer after surgical simulation training. *Ann Surg.* 2008;248:166–179.
22. Block EFJ, Lottenburg L, Flint L, et al. Use of a human patient simulator for the advanced trauma life support course. *Am Surg.* 2002;68:648.

23. Collicott PE. Advanced Trauma Life Support (ATLS): past, present, future, 16 Stone Lecture. *American Trauma Society: J Trauma*. 1992;35:749.
24. Aggarwal R, Crochet P, Dias A, et al. Development of a virtual reality training curriculum for laparoscopic cholecystectomy. *Br J Surg*. 2009;96:1086–1093.
25. Tang B, Hanna GB, Cuschieri A. Analysis of errors enacted by surgical trainees during skills training courses. *Surgery*. 2005;138(1):14–20.
26. Carter F, Russell E, Dunkley P, et al. Restructured animal tissue model for training laparoscopic anti-reflux surgery. *Min Invas Ther*. 1994;3:77–80.
27. Andreweatta PB, Woodrum DT, Dirkmeyer JD, et al. Laparoscopic skills are improved with LAP Mentor™ training: results of a randomized, double-blinded study. *Ann Surg*. 2006;243:854–860.
28. Aggrwal R, Boza C, Hance J, et al. Skills acquisition for laparoscopic gastric bypass in the training laboratory: an innovative approach. *Obes Surg*. 2007;17:19–27.
29. Meyerson SL, LoCascio F, Balderson SS, et al. An inexpensive, reproducible tissue simulator for teaching thoracoscopic lobectomy. *Ann Thorac Surg*. 2010:89:594–597.
30. Essani R, Scriven RJ, McLarty AJ, et al. Simulated laparoscopic sigmoidectomy training: responsiveness of surgery residents. *Dis Colon Rectum*. 2009;52:1956–1961.
31. The SH, Hunter JG, Sheppard BC. A suitable animal model for laparoscopic hepatic resection training. *Surg Endosc*. 2007;21:1738–1744.
32. Cundiff GW, Weidner AC, Visco AG. Effectiveness of laparoscopic cadaveric dissection in enhancing resident comprehension of pelvic anatomy. *J Am Coll Surg*. 2001;192:492–497.
33. Giger U, Fresard I, Hafliger A, et al. Laparoscopic training on Thiel human cadavers: a model to teach advanced laparoscopic procedures. *Surg Endosc*. 2008;22:901–906.
34. Barton DPJ, Davies DC, Mahadevan V, et al. Dissection of soft-preserved cadavers in the training of gynaecological oncologists: report of the first UK workshop. *Gynecologic Oncology*. 2009;113:352–356.
35. Levine RL, Kives S, Cathey G, et al. The use of lightly embalmed (fresh tissue) cadavers for resident laparoscopic training. *J Minim Invasive Gynecol*. 2006;13:451–456.
36. Schardey HM, Schopf S, Kammal M, et al. Invisible scar endoscopic thyroidectomy by the dorsal approach: experimental development of a new technique with human cadavers and preliminary clinical results. *Surg Endosc*. 2008;22:813–820.
37. Kohn LT, Corrigan JM, Donaldson MS. *To Err is Human*. Washington, DC: National Academies Press; 1999.

38. Leape LL, Brennan TA, Laird N, et al. The nature of adverse events in hospitalized patients: results of the Harvard Medical Practice Study II. *N Engl J Med.* 1991;324:377–384.
39. Thomas EJ, Studdert DM, Burstin HR, et al. Incidence and type of adverse events and negligent care in Utah and Colorado. *Med Care.* 2000;38:261–271.
40. Berwick DM. Errors today and errors tomorrow. *N Engl J Med.* 2003;348:2570–2572.
41. Gawande AA, Zinner MJ, Studdert DM, et al. Analysis of errors reported by surgeons at three teaching hospitals. *Surgery.* 2003;133:614–621.
42. Rogers SO, Jr, Gawande AA, Kwann M, et al. Analysis of surgical errors in closed malpractice claims at four liability insurers. *Surgery.* 2006;140:25–33.
43. Greenberg CC, Regenbogen SE, Struddert DM, et al. Patterns of communication breakdown resulting in injuries to surgical patients. *J Am Coll Surg.* 2007;204:533–540.
44. Lingard L, Espin S, Whyte S, et al. Communication failure in the operating room: an observational classification of recurrent types and effects. *Qual Saf Health Care.* 2004;13:330–334.
45. Healey MA, Shackford SR, Osler TM, Rogers FB, Burns E. Complications in surgical patients. *Arch Surg.* 2002;137:611–617.
46. Andrews LB, Stocking C, Krizek T, et al. An alternative strategy for studying adverse events in medical care. *Lancet.* 1997;349:309–313.
47. Yule S, Flin R, Paterson-Brown S, Maran N. Non-technical skills for surgeons in the operating room: a review of the literature. *Surgery.* 2006;139:140–149.
48. Hull L, Arora S, Aggarwal R, et al. The impact of non-technical skills on technical performance in surgery: a systematic review. *J Am Coll Surg.* 2012;214:214–230.
49. Martin JA, Regehr G, Reznick R, et al. Objective structured assessment of technical skills (OSATS) for surgical residents. *Br J Surg.* 1997;84: 273–278.
50. Aggarwal R, Grantcharov T, Moorthy K, et al. An evaluation of the feasibility, validity and reliability of laparoscopic skills assessment in the operating room. *Ann Surg.* 2007;245:992–999.
51. Spencer FC. Teaching and measuring surgical techniques: the technical evaluation of competence. *Bull Am Coll Surg.* 1978;63:9–12.
52. Flin R, Coeters K, Amalberti R, et al. The development of the NOTECHS system for evaluating pilots' CRM skills. *Human Factors and Aerospace Safety.* 2003;3:95–117.
53. Flin R, O'Connor P, Mearns K, et al. Crew resource management: training teams in high risk industries. *Team Performance Management.* 2002;8:68–78.

54. Fletcher GCL, McGeorge P, Flin RH, et al. The role of non-technical skills in anaesthesia: a review of current literature. *Br J Anaesth*. 2002;88: 418–429.
55. Aggarwal R, Undre S, Moorthy K, et al. The simulated operating theatre: comprehensive training for surgical team. *Qual Saf Health Care*. 2004;13:i27–i32.
56. Moorthy K, Munz Y, Adams S, et al. Human factors analysis of technical and team skills during procedural simulations. *Br J Surg*. 2003:90:88–89.
57. Mishra A, Catchpole K, McCulloch P. The Oxford NOTCHS System: reliability and validity of a tool for measuring teamwork behaviour in the operating theatre. *Qual Saf Health Care*. 2009;18;109–115.
58. Yule S, Flin R, Paterson-Brown S, et al. Development of a rating system for surgeons' non-technical skills. *Med Ed*. 2006;40:1098–1104.
59. Crossley J, Marriot J, Purdie H, et al. Prospective observational study to evaluate NOTSS (Non-Technical Skills for Surgeons) for assessing trainees' non-technical performance in the operating theatre. *Br J Surg*. 2011;98:1010–1020.
60. Undre S, Healey AN, Darzi A, et al. Observational assessment of surgical teamwork: a feasibility study. *World J Surg*. 2006;30:1774–1783.
61. Sharma B, Mishra A, Aggarwal R, et al. Non-technical skills assessment in surgery. *Surg Onc*. 2011;20:169–177.
62. Moorthy K, Munz Yaron, Forrest D, et al. Surgical crisis management skills training and assessment: a simulation-based approach to enhancing operating room performance. *Ann Surg*. 2006;244:139–147.
63. Powers K, Rehrig ST, Irias N, et al. Simulated laparoscopic operating room crisis: an approach to enhance the surgical team performance. *Surg Endosc*. 2008;22:885–900.
64. Holzman RS, Cooper JB, Gaba DM, et al. Anesthesia crisis resource management: real life simulation training in operating room crises. *J Clin Anesth*. 1995;7:675–687.
65. Moorthy K, Munz Y, Adams S, et al. A human factors analysis of technical and team skills among surgical trainees during procedural simulations in a simulated operating theatre. *Ann Surg*. 2005;242:631–639.
66. Park CS, Rochlen LR, Yaghmour E, et al. Acquisition of critical intraoperative event management skills in novice anesthesiology residents by using high-fidelity simulation-based training. *Anesthesiology*. 2010;112:202–211.

AUTHOR DETAILS

IRFAN AHMED FCPS, MD, FRCS
Senior Lecturer / Consultant Surgeon
Department Of Surgery
Aberdeen Royal Infirmary
Aberdeen, AB25 2ZN, UK

KAMRAN AHMED MBBS, MRCS, PhD
Guy's and St Thomas' NHS Foundation Trust
Urology Centre
Great Maze Pond
London, SE1 9RT, UK

RAJESH AGGARWAL MD, PhD, MA, FRCS
Instructor in Gastrointestinal Surgery
Department of Surgery
Perelman School of Medicine
University of Pennsylvania
3535 Market Street, Mezzanine
Philadelphia 19104, USA

ALI NEHME BAHSOUN BSc
Guy's and St Thomas' NHS Foundation Trust
Urology Centre
Great Maze Pond
London, SE1 9RT, UK

JAMES BREWIN FRCS(Urol)
Guy's and St Thomas' NHS Foundation Trust
Great Maze Pond
London, SE1 9RT, UK

BEN CHALLACOMBE MS, FRCS (Urol)
Guy's and St Thomas' NHS Foundation Trust
Urology Centre
Great Maze Pond
London, SE1 9RT, UK

PROKAR DASGUPTA MBBS, MSc(Urol), DLS, MD, FRCS, FRCS(Urol), FEBU
Chair in Robotic Surgery & Urological Innovation
Honorary Consultant Urological Surgeon
MRC Centre for Transplantation
NIHR Biomedical Research Centre
King's College London
5th Floor Tower Wing, Guy's Hospital
London, SE1 9RT, UK

JOHN FITZPATRICK MBChB
Academic Section of Urology
Medical Research Institute
Medical School, University of Dundee
Ninewells Hospital
Dundee, DD1 9SY, UK

DANIEL A. HASHIMOTO MD
Department of Biosurgery and Surgical Technology
St Mary's Hospital, Imperial College London
10th Floor Queen Elizabeth the Queen Mother Building
Praed Street, London, W2 1NY, UK

PETER JAYE
Simulation and Interactive Learning (SaIL) Centre
Guy's and St Thomas' NHS Foundation Trust
Great Maze Pond
London, SE1 9RT, UK

JEAN S. KER MbChB MD FRCPE FRCGP FHEA
Professor of Medical Education
Medical Education Institute
Schools of Medicine
College of Medicine, Dentistry and Nursing
Ninewells Hospital
Dundee, DD1 9SY, UK

FAHD KHAN MD, MRCS
Department of Urology
Darent Valley Hospital
Darenth Wood Road
Dartford, Kent, DA2 8DA, UK

MOHAMMED SHAMIM KHAN OBE, MBBS, MCPS, FRCS(Urol), FEBU
Guy's and St Thomas' NHS Foundation Trust
Urology Centre
Great Maze Pond
London, SE1 9RT, UK

NUZHATH KHAN BSc
Guy's and St Thomas' NHS Foundation Trust
Urology Centre
Great Maze Pond
London, SE1 9RT, UK

JASON Y. LEE MD, FRCSC
Assistant Clinical Professor
Division of Urology, Department of Surgery
St Michael's Hospital, University of Toronto
Associate Scientist, Keenan Research Centre
61 Queen St E – Suite 9-103
Toronto, Ontario, M5C 2T2, Canada

LARS LUND MD
Department of Urology
Odense University Hospital
Sdr Boulevard 29
5000 Odense C, Denmark

ELSPETH M. MCDOUGALL
MD, FRCSC, MHPE
Professor of Urology
Director, Surgical Education Center
Associate Dean, Simulation &
 Continuing Medical Education
Chair, AUA Office of Education
School of Medicine
University of California, Irvine
333 The City Blvd West, Suite 2100
Orange, CA 92868, USA

RAVINDRA MEHTA MBChB
Academic Section of Urology
Medical Research Institute
Medical School, University of
 Dundee
Ninewells Hospital
Dundee, DD1 9SY, UK

GHULAM NABI MS, MCh, MD, FTCS(Urol)
Senior Clinical Lecturer in Surgical
 Uro-oncology
and Hon. Consultant Urological
 Surgeon
Academic Section of Urology
Medical Research Institute
Medical School, University of
 Dundee
Ninewells Hospital
Dundee, DD1 9SY, UK

LAURA NICOL MRCS
Specialist Registrar
Department Of Surgery
Aberdeen Royal Infirmary
Aberdeen, AB25 2ZN, UK

JOHAN POULSEN MD
Department of Urology
Aalborg University Hospital
Hobrovej 18–22, Postboks 365
9100 Aalborg, Denmark

IAIN S. TAIT PhD FRCS
Department of Surgery and
 Cuschieri Skills Centre
Division of Clinical Academic
 Practice and Medical Education
 Institute
Ninewells Hospital and Medical
 School, University of Dundee
Dundee, DD1 9SY, UK

BENJIE TANG MD
Cuschieri Skills Centre
Medical Education Institute
Ninewells Hospital and Medical
 School, University of Dundee
Dundee, DD1 9SY, UK

HETTIE TILL MSc
MMedEd DEd
Lecturer in Assessment
Medical Education Institute
School of Medicine
College of Medicine, Dentistry and
 Nursing
Ninewells Hospital
Dundee, DD1 9SY, UK

SARAH WHEATSTONE
South London Healthcare NHS
 Foundation Trust
Frognal Avenue
Sidcup, Kent, DA14 6LT, UK